Moms Don't Get Sick

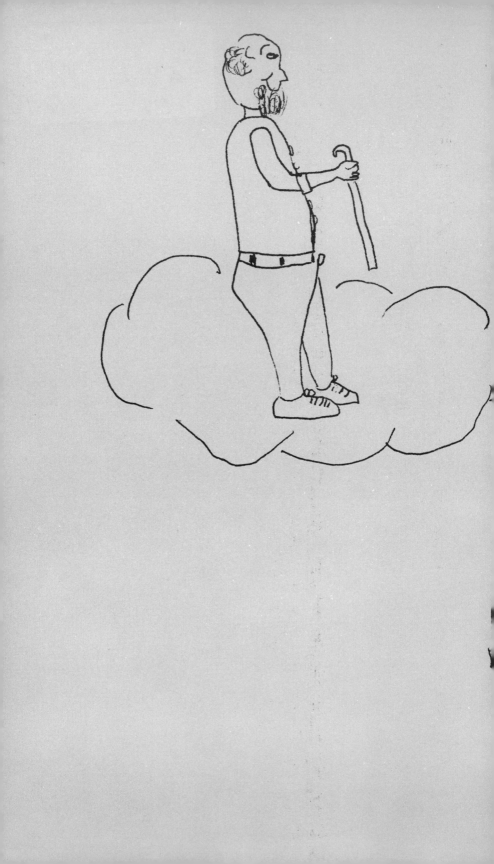

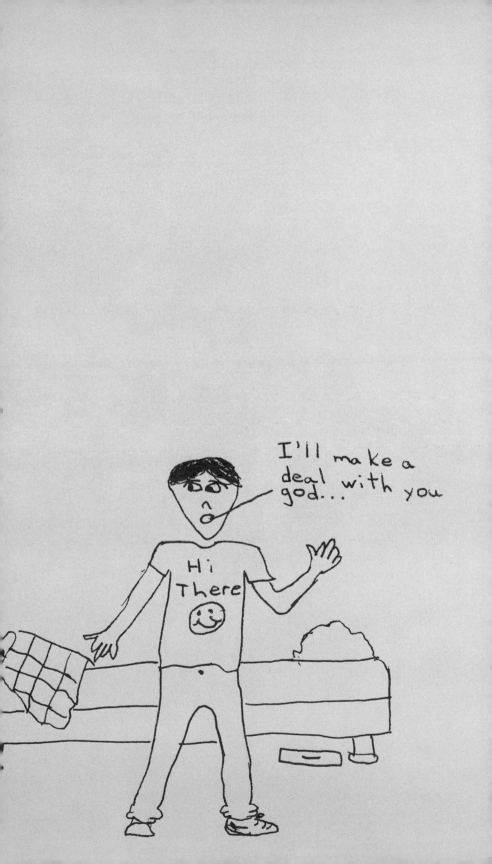

I Love her
I Love her
I Love her
I Love her r
I Love her
I Love her no
I Lovcher
I Love her r
I Love her!

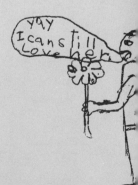

Moms Don't Get Sick

by *Pat Brack*
with Ben Brack

Illustrations by Ben Brack

MELIUS PUBLISHING CORPORATION

This Book Is Dedicated to the Person or Persons Who Visited Our Mailbox and Left Us the Courage to Keep Going.

While I was in the hospital recovering from my mastectomy I woke one night to find a little Christmas package at the foot of my bed. It was a beautiful little ornament of a partridge and a pear tree. It had no card and no one in the hospital knew how it had gotten there. Each night after that another gift appeared. When I got home the presents continued for each "day of Christmas." I got two red candles, three sprigs of holly, four red apples, five golden walnuts, six bows, seven gift tags and on to the twelfth day of Christmas with a dozen cookies. The whole family, especially Ben and I, would stake out the mailbox but never caught our secret Santa. On Christmas day we waited in vain for him/her/them to come by and reveal their identity but we never found out who it was. In the early days of my illness we spent much time plotting to catch this friend and trying to deduce who this angel could be. It helped. It was wonderful to have this magic to think about instead of the current horror show.

After Christmas the surprises in the mailbox continued. Every week some thoughtful present would arrive. My favorite shade of nail polish, a chocolate rose, spinach seeds for me to plant to help raise my low hematocrit, a medal for courage, bubble gum, a shamrock plant, an Easter basket, and, near the end of chemotherapy, barrettes for my new hair, a miniature of gin, sun block, and party invitations and balloons for my "coming out party." I still have no idea who drove to our remote country lane once every week for six months to leave these special gifts. I am not sure I want to know. I just want them to know what a difference it made looking forward to their visits and knowing that someone cared that much. Thank you.

Contents

ACKNOWLEDGEMENTS

We owe a warm thank you to many individuals who helped make this book possible.

First, our gratitude to Richard Hart for his hours of encouragement, editing, and literary expertise. Gerry Valerio, who used his time and talent in designing the book, gave all of us a timeless gift. Photographers Declan Haun and Butch Hodgson provided outstanding photos; Butch convinced Ben and me to stop clowning in front of his camera.

To our literary agent, Milly Marmur, who never stopped believing in our book, and special thanks to Ken Melius whose caring and thoughtful approach to its publication we appreciate more than we can say.

Our friends who cooked, chauffeured, held my hand, protected and listened: Helen and Roger Walters who spent almost as much time at the hospital as I did, Cheryl Hodgson, Sharie Valerio, Chrissi and Sebastian Zito, Patti Lahourcade, Ginny Bart, Alice Camara, Diana and Pat Rossello, Bud and Carolyn Howe, the Gathmanns, the Stones, the White Hall Russells, the Belfast Road Russells, Bart and Lois Evans, Rebecca Gilpin, Jenny and Raymond Lumley-Duchesne, Katy Lumley-Sapanski, the Keenans, the Barnes, Patience McPherson, Alicia Robards, Mary Kennedy, Esther Massengill, Diane Proctor, Brad Marshall, the Selways and the Hardys, Asa and Sue Erickson, we cherish your support.

My medical SWAT team, Dr. Victor Khousami who got me to the right doctors at the right time, Dr. Bernard McGibbon who was always there to put things back together, Dr. Charles

Padgett who continues to keep our show on the road, and
Adil Totoonchie whose surgical skill paradoxically kept me wl
The warm competence of these people and all the others at Gre
Baltimore Medical Center made a bad situation tolerable. A
my appreciation for my support group NEED, you were t
when I needed you.

The faculty, staff, students and parents at Ruxton Cou
School who believed in my survival and helped me pull it
especially Sally Wilkes, Judy Banker, Joan Owens, Bar
Grossman who introduced us to Milly, MaryJo Fitzgibbons, I
Hawley, Robin Lenci, George Rayburn, Mary Lou Hanley
Carol Kotras, and Barbara Smith.

I'm thankful for the increased closeness with my sister,
D'Zmura, who helped us through Christmas, confusion, and ch
by understanding and doing my shopping for me.

Last, I want to say thank you to my family, whose existe
humor and perception made it all worthwhile.

INTRODUCTION

Having a parent become seriously ill causes unexpected change and confusion within a family. To have the family optimist and comforter out of commission is a major shock to a child. *Moms Don't Get Sick* is the true story of a ten-year-old, Ben, and me, his mother, who for all of his life had been a strong, funny and seemingly consistent part of his existence.

When it was found that I had breast cancer, life changed for our family suddenly and dramatically. This book chronicles the events and feelings experienced by Ben and me as we struggled to adapt to this new situation and salvage our close relationship.

The book and its title were Ben's idea. He thought that no child should ever have to go through this experience and, by sharing his story, he might be able to help someone else. (That he might become famous was another consideration.) That both Ben and I could begin to have some peace about it is an added bonus. We have tried to give an honest account of our pain and emotional survival. In my case, so far, the long term prognosis is good. Nonetheless Ben and I explored the possibility that survival is not always possible: recognizing that death is sometimes a premature reality is part of the strengthening for parent and child.

The book begins from Ben's perspective as he describes our family and the crisis as he remembers it. His observations are followed by my narrative as I attempt to "fill in" factual detail, setting, and the chronology of the events taking place. Both voices express our initial confusion, pain, and our sometimes misguided

attempts to communicate, cope and help each other through
unfairly difficult time.

Moms Don't Get Sick uses tape recorded intervi
conversations and entries which I kept in a journal during
course of my surgeries, chemotherapy and recovery. As Ben
it, "I spoke; you wrote." We went through all the classic s
of grief: denial, depression, anger, bargaining, alienation,
acceptance. These stages are shared not only in their terri
aspects but with humor and irony as both Ben and I reacte
family members tend to do, at cross purposes and with n
signals. Some of our bungled attempts to communicate
only understood when Ben and I were in the process of ta
and taping the interviews (for which I might add, Ben cha
$1.00 per hour—our budding entrepreneur).

The specific disease in our story is breast cancer, and v
definitions, problems and treatment are discussed, it is dor
part of the narrative and is not meant to document this parti
disease. The focus of the book is rather to describe the difficu
involved for both parents and children when any major h
problem invades a family.

Moms Don't Get Sick deals primarily with the relatior
between Ben and me during this period. Ben had just turnec
when the cancer was discovered. Too old to be oblivious tc
turmoil around him and too young to have a support sy
other than his family, he was the most vulnerable of all o
Our teenage sons, Jeb and Sean, while scared and saddene
the unexpected turn of events, were both in that stage of
where they were wrapped up in what was happening in
own lives. Jeb had just left home to begin his freshman ye
college and Sean, though living at home, had begun the pro
of breaking away from the family group to become immerse
rock music and his friends. He helped whenever he coulc
was there to comfort me and give me a hug when I badly ne
it. He had, however, developed ways of coping that Ben, t
much younger, had not.

My husband Bill was left to pick up all the pieces dro
by the rest of us when my illness was diagnosed. Carpools, m

shopping, kid's homework, bills, and insurance forms all had to be juggled as he tried to manage his own job and our house and provide all of us with the reassurance we badly needed. I don't know how he did it; I secretly feel that as bad as cancer was, having to be the strong one for everyone and fearing that you might lose your best friend would be worse. He not only had to pick up the pieces, he also had to pretend for all of us that things were under control. Bill is here in the book; he is the constant support that allowed Ben and me to have the energy to help each other and eventually to put our story in print. He did everything he could for all of us. He still does.

Our family has been crying, hugging, yelling, laughing, and healing ever since. Our perception and appreciation of each other has been forever changed. Child has become more adult and adult has regained both the joy and some of the selfishness of childhood. By sharing our story we hope others may find some recognition that we are similar in our darker moments and, by sharing, we can provide hope and perhaps help for our readers. Illness changes us and it hurts; it can also help us gain new strength and a renewed appreciation of what we once took for granted.

PAT BRACK

Moms Don't Get Sick

The World Turned Upside Down

Mothers are the people who make sure you drink your milk and make you wear a raincoat even if it's just cloudy. They are important to a kid because they remember where you are supposed to be. They keep things going. I realized just how important they are two years ago when my mom got cancer. Thinking my mom might die was the worst thing that had ever happened to me. It seemed like, up until then, I'd had a perfect childhood. All of my life, at least the part I can remember, I have lived in a big old farmhouse in the country with narrow winding stairways and lots of doors to make it great for hide-and-seek. I've had a barn with a loft to jump out of or use as a clubhouse, huge old trees to climb and rest in and lanes with no cars where I can ride my bike. Jeb and Sean, my big brothers, were older when we moved out here and they remember living in the city. They missed some things like being able to walk to stores or the library. Now they like living in the country, but when they talk about the old days, they talk about neighborhood gangs and back yards. Mom and Dad grew up in the city too. They had always had this dream of a big garden and lots of space, so when I wasn't even one year old, we all moved to the country.

It must have been really strange for all of them to suddenly live off by ourselves. I think it made us closer to each other as we sometimes didn't have other people to talk to or play with. I do know that we seem to have a lot of traditions and things that we do together so that we don't get lonely. We have lots of picnics

and parties at our house to share the country with our frie
We have celebrations for almost every holiday. We "trici
treat" at Halloween in the car because the houses are so far a
We get lots of stuff at each place because people don't see n
kids in costumes and they invite you in. They are so glad tc
you. Some neighbors dress up and have scary lights and sou
It is neat.

At Christmas our house looks just like a Christmas
especially when it snows. We have candles in the windows
wreaths on all the doors. The house fills with packages
friends. We read Christmas stories together, and we bake fc
gingerbread people and decorate them like famous people. W
had Dolly Parton, Bob Hope and even Richard Nixon on
tree.

We have a certain way we always put up the tree. It is alu
too big for the corner and Mom makes us move it over and
until it is straight. We have this terrible record of Christ
carols that Mom bought from the gas station long ago.
hates it and complains every year. We play it anyway as we
the tree and Dad threatens to burn it. We have made tape co
in case he ever does. Dad has bought some new beautiful Christ
music but we still play that old record. It is part of what
always do.

I can't imagine living anywhere else. I like the wide o
spaces for star watching and flashlight tag. I love looking
my bedroom window and surprising a family of deer eating
grapes. Our fields are full of rabbits, chipmunks and sna
mostly non-poisonous. I love them all. Living in the cour
seems just right to me.

PAT: Moving to the country was a daring decision for Bill, my husba
and me. Both of us had grown up in city neighborhoods, master
bus routes, double-locking our doors, and outwitting poten
muggers for much of our lives. We wanted something differ
for our family and when Ben, our third child and a comp
surprise, entered the picture we had to decide between moving
a larger house in the city or retreating past the suburbs to

fantasy of rural life where cows and sheep outnumber people. I still recall the fear I had at leaving my pediatrician so far behind, not to mention city water and sewage systems, walking to the grocery store, and easily available babysitters. Still we decided to do it.

We moved Sean, a six-year-old herpetologist, an extremely skeptical ten-year-old, Jeb, who would have preferred a high rise apartment, and our baby, Ben, who was just learning to walk and was ready for the adventures of electric fences and cows which occasionally got loose and wandered through our front yard.

The house proved to be a challenge from the start. A "sweat equity" farmhouse, it has been a treasure and constant source of frustration for over ten years. The house was a run-down, Victorian-style sitting on three acres of land and was visually, if one ignored two or three tons of scrap metal and trash, the embodiment of the simple country life.

Amid rusting cans and peeling paint stood a frame house complete with leaky roof, rotting porch and early American plumbing. Around the ghastly remains of an above-ground swimming pool stood six old apple trees (surely qualifying as an orchard) and a ruined grape arbor. Finally there were outbuildings, the ultimate distinguishing feature between rural and suburban.

We took on the Herculean task of transforming our find into a home. For months we worked, disposing of a quarter century's collection of trash. We sanded floors, peeled multiple layers of old wallpaper from cracked plaster walls, installed new plumbing and a septic system and tried to beat back years of untended landscaping. All of this was done beneath the skeptical gaze of our city-bred children, who announced that the place smelled bad (it did) and that it would be much more fun to go to a movie.

After ten years the house still creaks and the pump occasionally quits when someone is fully soaped in the shower. There is one room, the kitchen, where we can be toasty warm in winter, thanks to the presence of a wood stove. In spring the grass still grows too quickly and powdery mildew has been known to invade our orchard.

Our family has grown up here. We have gone through pe
of sons' adopting snakes for pets and through graduation
birthday parties for family and friends. We have even ha
sad privilege of burying a good friend's ashes in our garden

We love the welcoming bay windows which draw peop
rather than shut them out. We always have a feeling of pr
but never isolation. I have a big farm kitchen where we can
bread and spread it with jam from our own grapes. Chil
my own and their friends, come here to launch model roc
have massive water gun battles, climb trees, and form secret soc
in the loft of the barn.

Our boys, nineteen, seventeen, and ten are growing up
diverse and enjoyable human beings. This description admit
facts that no one mows the lawn without being asked repea
and, who does the dishes (and has the most onerous part) rer
a nightly debate even after ten years of KP duty. They still
for my husband Bill and me to fold under the pressure and
them all out of the kitchen. We rarely do.

The children have had their share of academic difficul
have spent more than fifteen years sitting across the desk
various teachers being told that my children have excellent m
but need to learn to apply themselves. They seem more inter
in making people laugh than in doing school work. Somet
the same child will be reported as withdrawn. None of my offs
have ever viewed homework as a reasonable obligation.

The boys' rooms are minefields of dirty clothing and disca
partially completed projects from term papers to models of med
castles or the World Trade Center. The ambience is a ble
loud rock music and unmade beds. They are designed specifi
to discourage adult visitors. The older boys also demand
birthright the ownership of an automobile and the issuanc
their sixteenth birthday of a driver's license. Their expecta
are not always realized. On occasion they reprimand us, li
in great detail and with precision our failings, broken pro
and our utter and total unreasonableness. In short, from w
hear from our straightforward friends, we are a run-of-the
normal family.

We have been happy living in the country. It has been a safe place. It was not a place for serious illness to intrude.

Mothers are the ones who make sure you have your school supplies each fall. They notice you've grown over the summer and that your sneakers have holes and no laces. They take care of those things.

Mothers don't always hang around baking cookies anymore. A lot of them have jobs and get cranky and tired of fixing dinner and telling you to do your homework. But they are there and they do go to P.T.A. and they do tuck you in at night. You know they are in charge.

Most of the time the worst thing that happens to your mom is she gets a cold or the flu and goes to bed. The shopping has to be done by Dad and the house gets really messy, which doesn't bother anyone but Mom anyway. Soon she gets better and begins to boss the family around about picking up socks and underwear. Things are back to normal.

One day normal changed at our house. My mom went to the doctor. When she got home she looked pale and serious. She didn't say much to me and spent a lot more time than usual on the phone. When Dad got home he and Mom went off together and talked so that I couldn't hear much. I don't remember getting a real dinner that night.

Mom and Dad told us kids that Mom had to go to a specialist for some tests but not to worry, it probably wasn't anything too serious. I felt puzzled; what was going on here? No one seemed to know I was there. Usually our family blurts out everything that goes wrong. This time Mom and Dad were too quiet.

The next few days were not like our house at all. Dad looked like he had been crying. I had never seen my dad look like that. Mom and Dad said that Mom had to go to the hospital but not to worry, it was probably okay. They didn't look like it was probably okay.

While Mom was in the hospital, friends of the family and my friends were really nice to me. I got to sleep over at a friend's house on a school night and my teachers didn't check my homework

*as carefully as usual. I kind of liked the attention but I
little guilty about mom. Not too guilty though, because I
the hospital would fix her up.*

PAT: The discovery that almost certainly I had cancer was the
disruptive event of my entire life. Within hours my world
had known it dissolved and was replaced by the immediate prob
of how severe my condition was, what treatment was avai
and what tests should be done when. My emotional reac
were a bit slow. At first I couldn't believe it at all, then as
evidence accrued, Bill and I had to make critical decisions
in a state of shock and disbelief.

After a decisive morning with the radiologist (he said
mammogram and other tests confirmed an eighty percent ch
of a malignancy), I immediately headed for the nearest shop
mall to buy the children everything in sight. My rationaliza
for this—and it turned out to be accurate—was that if I
cancer diagnosed in early December, this would seriously a
my Christmas shopping time. Christmas has always been
time at our house, mostly engineered by me. If I was o
commission, I couldn't imagine how it would happen.

I still remember walking zombielike from store to store fi
shopping bags in a desperate effort to restore some illusio
sanity to life.

This frantic effort was soon replaced by the arrangement
my hospitalization and numerous consultations in which I
to learn all I could about a disease I, by choice, knew very
about. Bill and I tried to communicate with the children du
those hectic days but were so unsure of things ourselves that
afraid the discussions were more hollow reassurances than
real attempt to share what was happening with the boys. "Th
are under control," we said, "the doctors will be able to fix th
up. You can help by doing the dishes without fighting and gi
us some quiet time . . ."

It is hard to respond to children when you, the patient,
in the denial stage of a medical crisis. Add to this the worl
medicine and its technology, which I find completely overwh

me. I gave in to it. I emotionally deserted my family as I entered this new and confusing actuality.

When Mom came home from the hospital after her first trip she had to rest most of the time. People brought food and flowers and came to visit. Mom and Dad gave us a VCR as an early Christmas present and we watched a lot of movies. Only Mom kept falling asleep.

Finally Mom told me that what she had was cancer of her breast and that she had to go back to the hospital for more surgery (that means cutting out the cancer). She said that she hoped she'd be okay after this operation. She didn't sound very sure and I didn't want to ask too many questions. I was beginning to wish that this was a tape for the new VCR and I could just rewind it to before all this started. I wanted our old life back. But it was no go. This was really happening.

On the first trip to the hospital I had a lumpectomy, a surgical procedure used to remove the tumor and some surrounding tissue. The hope is that the tumor is encapsulated and that the rest of the breast can be saved.

Waking up in the recovery room following surgery, I was told that, as strongly suspected, the tumor was malignant and, worse news, that there was no definitive area within the breast where the cancer cells stopped. A modified radical mastectomy was recommended. This procedure involves removing the entire breast and a number of lymph nodes from under the arm so that pathologists can determine if and how much the cancer cells have spread. The situation seemed to be getting worse at a very fast pace. I struggled to overcome the effects of the general anesthesia as I tried to assimilate this latest disaster. It seemed I was to be sent home for five days to contemplate my fate while the pathologists prepared more extensive studies and my further surgery could be scheduled. I felt I had fallen into the "Twilight Zone."

To watch one's family struggle with the shock of learning that Mom is *really* sick was one of the hardest parts of the illness for me. The word "cancer" is so scary and suddenly Mom as the

comforter, the hugger, the one whose optimism is suppose
make things all right is gone. Kaput. Out of commissior
couldn't say, "It'll be okay." My personal rug had been pu
out from under me and I was terrified and not sure of anytl

I'd watch the pale, concerned faces of my family and be un
to give any reassurance. I would watch my childrens' lives b
uprooted and twisted and know that this cancer in me was destro
something in them. Things I'd tried for years to nurture v
being undermined. Stability for example, security, and innoce
And my illness was at fault.

BEN: *Christmas was very near and none of the special things i*
happening at our house. My mom does bake at Christmas, gi
bread boys, special bread and tollhouse cookies. Weeks be
Christmas packages and wrappings start filling the house. It
wasn't happening that year.

My mom was in the hospital again. I went to see her t
after her operation. Her room was full of these red Chris
flowers. Mom was in a bed that had buttons to make the i
or foot go up and down. She had a light, a television, a ph
and an intercom you could work from the bed. I hopped u,
the bed and everyone said, "Sit still, be careful, don't bounc

I couldn't really even hug her as she had this big ban
with tubes and little drain bags hanging from them. Still
helped me figure out a way to snuggle with her and she le
work the buttons and she shared her candy.

I didn't like having Mom there. It was like the hospital ou
her and she wasn't really my mother anymore. I wanted he
come home with us right then. She said she couldn't come i
the hospital thought she was well enough. She looked sad
said that she wanted to come home more than anything. I d
know what to do so I started acting kind of silly and ran in
halls. I hated that place. I finally hid under a chair and
all, even Mom, had to look for me. I was mad at all of th
Even though it wasn't Mom's fault, I was angry. The whole t
just wasn't fair.

Returning to the hospital required some courage on my part. This trip I remembered what surgery felt like. Fortunately I spent much of that time in a foggy state where I accepted, for the most part, what I had to do. It was not unlike going into a final exam in college; you've done all you could to prepare for it, now it must be left to the gods to sort things out.

Waking up the second time after surgery was not too bad; I'd gone in knowing what to expect and felt a certain gratitude that I was waking up at all. Tubes, IVs, drains and some pain seemed to be the order of the day, but most of all, I felt relief that the cancer had been cut out and that the worst was over. I was surviving. People gathered bringing flowers, food, and stuffed animals and I enjoyed being the center of attention. I allowed myself the forgotten luxury of childhood: other people were in charge. I watched my remote control TV whenever I wanted to, I ate whatever came in on trays that I hadn't prepared. I entertained, enjoyed myself and amazed my visitors with my wonderful positive attitude.

We waited to bring Ben in for a visit until some time had passed and I had the strength to reassure him. He walked in looking for his mother and found this rather fragile, self-involved person who had in the past few weeks relegated motherhood to a back burner. I rallied to the point of sharing my bed and figuring out how to hold him without hurting too much. I felt the first stirring of panic that eventually I would be expected to resume the roles I had temporarily abandoned. It didn't seem fair. I had enough to work on: getting my left arm mobile again, having stitches and staples removed, and most of all, defining who I was, this person who had cancer.

My life now was divided into two parts. "B.C." was life before cancer; "A.C." was anything that happened to me from now on. I couldn't remember much about the time before cancer; I wondered why I hadn't been happier then. I wanted to see if I could figure out a way to return to that innocence when good health is a given. Instead the pathology report came back with the bad news that I had lymph node involvement, which meant

that some cancerous cells had spread from the breast and c
be lurking almost anywhere in my body.

Immediately, I had to have more tests to see if any vital or
were involved. Even more unthinkable to me, I had to con
the prospect of chemotherapy, a treatment about which I'd h
and of which I was terrified.

I wanted some time away to think this through before I v
home to my family. Unfortunately the modern hospital is no
up to handle this part of a patient's recovery and, after six d
a week before Christmas, the drains and I were released to re
the family.

BEN: *Mom came home right before Christmas. She was very u
so other people baked cookies for us and Dad cooked the tur
My brothers put up wreaths and garlands and Mom came downs
to put a few ornaments on the tree. It was a little strange bec
no one fought over the lights or where the decorations should
I was worried that the secret special things that Mom doe
Christmas wouldn't happen. She just seemed so tired and no
excited about the holidays as she always had been before.*

*When Christmas morning finally arrived it was great ar
even forgot that Mom had cancer. We all got up early like
always do and went downstairs to the stacks of presents pilea
a beautiful tree. I got a Lego castle which I really wanted
my brother Jeb and I started building it right away. Friends c
bringing more presents and we had a wonderful turkey dir
with stuffing and Christmas pudding. I felt so happy that I jum
on Mom to give her a huge bear hug. Everybody said "N
and made me stop. I can still feel my ears turning red and
body going all hot inside. Mom looked so sad. Things were
back to normal after all.*

PAT: The recent findings about adjuvant chemotherapy—that
chemotherapy given when no active tumor can be found but can
cells have been found outside the site of the tumor—indicate
it is best to begin the course of treatment as soon as possible a
surgery and in fairly aggressive doses. In addition to my surge

my gynecologist, and my radiologist, I acquired an oncologist, or cancer specialist, Dr. Padgett. He carefully explained the treatment to me and would have had me on my shots on Christmas Day had I not pointed out that the 25th is a fairly important holiday. Instead, two days after my release from the hospital, I was in Dr. Padgett's office preparing for this further trauma to my weary body and confused psyche. My treatments involved an IV push of two strong anticancer drugs, Methotrexate and 5-Fluorouracil. This was administered for two sessions a week apart, plus a daily oral dose of four Cytoxan tablets each morning for two weeks. This regimen would be followed by a two-week "off" period to give the body and its white and red cell counts an opportunity to rebuild themselves for the next round. This pattern for me was to continue for the next six months.

I reacted in the classic way to the medications: I threw up after the IV drugs and felt terrible after the pills. For the next two weeks I could take my Cytoxan, waking early to enjoy an hour or two without the queasiness I knew would return once I swallowed my pills.

At Christmas I'd had only one IV treatment and a few days of Cytoxan. I felt tired but full of gratitude that I was being given some treatment that gave me a better chance to survive. I was filled with the desire to produce as much holiday tradition and fun as I possibly could. Friends came by and wrapped the gifts I'd acquired on my frantic shopping trip. The family decorated and carried on, anxious to create a Christmas as usual. The feast appeared and all of us present felt how precious these times together are. Then, poor Ben, his natural exuberance restored, threw himself at me and realized that one of his Christmas wishes hadn't come true. He wanted his old mother back. She couldn't make it yet. Both of us hurt.

Bad Gets Worse

During the holidays Mom told me she had to start chemotherapy. This is a treatment for cancer where the doctor gives you very strong medicines that go into your blood and all over your body to kill cancer cells. Mom tried to explain that some cells are fighter cells, kind of like Luke Skywalker, and that cancer cells are bad cells attacking like Darth Vader in Star Wars. My family tried to explain how this works, but I got very confused. There are red blood cells and there are white blood cells and they are both good. If there are not the right number of cells, people can get sick.

Chemotherapy helps fight the bad cells, the cancer cells, but sometimes it kills good cells by accident also. This can make the person taking the medicine feel very tired and sicker than they seemed to be without the chemotherapy. It was all confusing to me and to Mom too. We are used to medicine making you feel better right away. It seemed funny that this medicine can make you feel worse before it makes you feel better.

So, Mom got chemotherapy and would throw up a lot. She spent a lot of time in bed and we would have to keep our radios turned way down.

No one was in charge in our house. Dad had to go to work and do so many of the jobs that Mom should have been doing. Mom kept trying to go to work and she would come home too tired to talk or help with my homework. I felt so helpless; I should have been able to change things, be a hero, but I didn't know how. Dad would yell at me in this voice, "DO THE KITCHEN, YOUR ROOM IS A MESS, HOMEWORK!!!"

Sometimes I would try very hard to be nice to Mom an
run errands for her and get her cold drinks. Some other tir
thought she should just get up and stop being lazy. So I u
yell at her. That didn't work either. She'd just look pale
maybe cry a little.

PAT: Chemotherapy for me was an unpleasant and debilitating pro
Constantly exhausted and feeling ill, I had a difficult time convin
myself that this was indeed giving me a much better sh(
survival. In order to keep going I'd make lists of reasor
survive; the good things. This was sometimes ludicrous, as r
of my "good things" that I most cared about became increas
sullen and unhappy. Still winter passed and we all carried

I remember that Easter came early that year. Easter
important occasion in our lives, not so much for its relig
significance, but because our country location is an ideal
for an Easter egg hunt. It is the first picnic of spring.
though Easter usually coincides with mud season, it mean
have survived the winter. That a chilly rain frequently force:
picnic indoors does not dampen our belief that the worst o
winter is past and that daffodils will bloom again.

I wanted so much to keep our traditions, to live life a
always had. It wasn't happening. I was too tired. So Easte
Brack rite of spring, moved elsewhere. Still Easter was fu
found an abandoned bird's nest in the barn and filled it
robin's egg candy. I bought a silly little mechanical bird wh
on top of the nest. For Ben I compromised my ethics and i
and got him a G.I. Joe figure he had wanted for months. T(
a "Cobra Ninja" in an Easter basket seemed the worst kir
hypocrisy, but I was glad to be able to give the child somet
anything, that would make him happy. Besides, I bought lc
little chicks and flowery items to atone.

Easter that year was glorious. We planted a pussy w
and began, as an act of faith, a perennial garden. The w
family pitched in: turning earth, adding peat moss, planting flo
Flowers grew. I spent time, often with a young helper, wee

and fussing in the new garden imagining masses of exotic bloom. Spring crept up on us all. I guess I hadn't expected it.

Exhaustion was the primary side effect I felt from the treatment. I tried to keep working and arranged a reduced schedule during the six months of therapy. Still I was always tired.

For the first time since I'd become a mother I had to put aside time for me, denying what most children feel are their unassailable rights. P.T.A. meetings fell by the wayside, bake sale requests were ignored. Car pools and the activities they entailed were dropped. Dinner was usually managed late by Bill after a full day of work. The children's schoolwork was either done by them or not done. Our sixteen-year-old used this as a marvelous opportunity to lower his grades. As I had always been the principal nagger about picking up, cleaning rooms and putting dirty laundry in baskets, the family became confused. There was no one who had the energy to bitch at them. The house got very dirty. At rare times people would clean the bathroom without being asked. There are minor victories that help one survive the major battles.

Sometimes school was horrible while Mom was sick. Most of the teachers acted like nothing had happened to Mom or to me and I had to pretend that my life at home was normal. My teacher still sent notes home when I acted up and I was kind of glad about that. It made me feel that I was a regular member of the class.

Still I knew that everyone knew about Mom. Some of the boys would tease me about how my mother was going to die. One of them would sing that horrible song about "The worms crawl in, the worms crawl out, the ants play pinochle on your snout." It is all about what happens to dead bodies. I had to pretend it didn't bother me. I have always been a kind of noisy kid but I got even noisier that year. I'd try to get other people in trouble and make silly noises to get people to laugh.

One person, the guidance counselor, would talk to me sometimes and that helped. I knew she and Mom had talked and that I could say anything to her and she wouldn't tell anyone else. My old third grade teacher would ask me how Mom was doing and

that made me feel better. My good friends would mayb*
"Imsorryaboutyourmom" real fast and I'd say "Okay" be*
none of us wanted to talk about it. It was too embarrassir

Girls were better friends when Mom was sick. They u*
say right out how hard it must be for me. They would as*
questions and I knew they really cared about how I was fe*
Girls can show they care and it doesn't make them look ba*

Mom tried to make our house seem normal some of the*
and would invite my friends over. Most of the time it just a*
seem right. I hated it when my friends were there and my*
was in bed or throwing up. I didn't like being different and *
the only one with a sick mother.

One time, though, I had my friend Robin over. We hac*
big project to do for our reading class. We were making a mini*
house and we needed to use flour, sugar, glitter, glue and all *
of little things. We destroyed Mom's kitchen and she didn't*
get mad. Robin and I really had fun and we both got an*
for our project.

After Robin went home, Mom and I talked about wh*
super day it had been. For that time, things had seemed like*
used to be. Then Mom asked me to put my slippers on bec*
it was chilly and I said "No." She couldn't believe it and I*
kept saying "No." She started to scream at me and I starte*
go upstairs. A little of the way up, I whispered, "Shut up."*
Mom heard and totally lost her temper. She picked me up*
shook me and said she'd be dipped in chocolate before any*
told her to shut up. She backed me up and held me to the*
and told me that I would do exactly what she told me to do*
ELSE!! I went and got my slippers on fast. I felt better th*
had in a long time. I think now that I back-talked on pur*
to see if Mom was really in there. She sure was and that r*
me feel warm and safer. Later we hugged and made up. It*
a wonderful day.

PAT: I remember so clearly the "slipper" episode and my fury at*
when he defied me and muttered, "Shut up." In that incohe*
moment I realized how little discipline he'd been getting fron*

and how far I had let things slide. Energy born of rage and frustration took hold and I decided I would rather die instantly of over-exertion than watch this once-lovable boy become an obnoxious little beast. A battle ensued. I found untapped energy enough to bounce him about the house. He later told me that I'd make a good goalie for his soccer team.

After this volcanic encounter, Ben put on his slippers and became very cheerful and loving. I think children need to feel that someone other than themselves is in control. Even though he had had a lovely day with a friend, or perhaps because he had had such a special day, I think he was worried that he'd gotten away with too much and needed to make sure that he still had a mother.

Both of us were shocked, surprised and relieved to find that bits of her "old self" remained and that limits, however shaky they had become, still existed.

When Mom wasn't too sick she would make jokes that helped a lot. I felt that things weren't as hopeless when she could laugh and when she would let me tease her about it. She let me see her scar and it wasn't nearly as bad as I had imagined. It was strange to see her with a part missing, but she was still Mom. I remember when she got her prosthesis, which is a false bosom, that she would put into her bra so that her clothes would look better. She'd let me toss it around. It felt like a water balloon, and I even tried it on to make my mother laugh. Mom said that she had a friend who even named her prosthesis "Fred," but Mom didn't want to get that attached to hers because she was planning to have an operation to do what doctors call "reconstruction." This means they operate and somehow make the two sides match again.

As chemotherapy went on, my mother lost almost all of her hair. I remember she would joke about it. Like how she woke up one morning and thought there was a new dog sleeping on her pillow. Then she realized it wasn't a new dog at all; it was her hair.

After most of Mom's hair fell out she bought a wig. I t
I hated that most of all the changes in our lives. She just d
look like my mom at all. It was too wavy and thick, too f.
Mom's face looked pale and small inside the wig and it sc
me. She looked like one of those fake people in a store win
only sick. Mom didn't like it either because she didn't we
very long. She switched to pretty scarves. She looked much b
then.

PAT: Losing my hair was one of the most humiliating parts of
entire bout with cancer. The mind is trying to cope with phy
losses, pain and the chilling reality that one is mortal. The l
is trying to adjust to a whole new terrain, and a series of
and frightening side effects from both surgery and treatn
Burning eyes, mouth sores, swelling around the surgical area
arm, bloating, and irregular heartbeats are some of the symp
people must deal with, varying from patient to patient.

It is a lot. I had decided to act out, as much as possible
charade of normalcy during my treatment. With the help
well fitted prosthesis, I could look natural.

Then the hair falls out. In my case, having thick hair, it
a while and I kept hoping I'd hit maximum thinning and it w
stop. I invested in a "Liza Minnelli pixie type" hair cut reaso
that thin hair looks better short and if I was to lose all my
I'd rather have it fall on the floor of the hair salon than on
pillow.

The head has many more hairs than we realize. Espec
when handful by handful they land on the floor of your sho
One chilly day in early March my scalp burned and hurt a
saw the truth. I was, while not totally bald, more scalp than
Something had to be done.

Wig shopping under such circumstances is not a fun tri
ended up with an expensive wig that had far too much hair.
family, while trying to be supportive and understanding, felt
I was somehow just not me, that this wig was out of chara
It was. I've always had relatively short hair that I showered
the rest of me and did little else about. Now I looked perpetu

as though I'd just had a professional set from Dolly Parton's stylist. Such irony. Worse yet, the thing made my scalp itch and I would absentmindedly scratch, leaving the blasted wig at various strange angles on my head.

Finally there was the philosophy of the wig. Damn it, I'd been sick. I'd lost a breast, my sense of well-being and now, my hair. It was time to begin to live with all this, to learn to accept this new self with all the changes. So I didn't have hair. I discovered scarves and the fun of playing gypsy. I bought and borrowed a complete wardrobe of them and created outfits with coordinating country cotton bandannas or sophisticated silks. Ben and I would sort them out to decide what costume to dream up for a special occasion. Blending fantasy and reality, it was fun to play dress-up.

The Whistler's Mother

The word "cancer" has an ugly, scary sound. It seems like grown-ups always know someone who has it and they talk about it in a soft, serious voice. For a long time no one in our family wanted even to say the word. Mom helped us there. She would come right out and say "Cancer." She would say the word cancer so often that it got boring. She'd say "Ben, build a fire and warm this room; your mother has cancer" or "What do you mean you didn't do your homework; your mother has cancer?" After awhile, especially when she was silly about it, the word didn't seem as horrible and we began to say it without that cold nasty feeling each time. When you can say it often enough, it takes away some of the fear.

Still I didn't want to talk about it very much. My mom and dad would try to explain things about it but most of the time I wouldn't really listen. I know now that this was a big mistake and made things harder for Mom and me.

For one thing I thought that cancer was contagious. The only sicknesses I knew about were colds, flu, chicken pox, lice, and maybe measles. Every time somebody is sick, the parents won't let you play together. They say, "Keep away from Joey, you'll catch his cold" or something like that. I didn't see that cancer should be any different and no one told me I couldn't catch it.

So, I began staying away from Mom as much as I could; at least I didn't hug and kiss her like I always had before. When Dad, Mom and I would snuggle for a story, I'd turn my head away from her so she couldn't breathe cancer germs on me. I was surprised that so many friends came to see her, I thought

they must be afraid too. I kept waiting for the rest of the f
and some of our friends to catch it. It wasn't until now
Mom and I were talking about all this that I finally foun
the truth. Cancer is not contagious. Many diseases are no
I could have saved myself a lot of trouble by asking about
also wouldn't have hurt Mom's feelings by turning my head
so often. If one of your parents comes down with a serious il
it is better to learn as many facts as you can about their dis
Not knowing does not make them any better and you can
some fearful times that you don't have to have. Keeping fe
yourself is a bad idea. I've learned now that I'd rather kno
the truth. Even if it is bad, my imagination can make it w

PAT: As I have been a teacher for most of my adult life, I sl
have had the knowledge and the skill to talk about cancer to
who is exactly the same age as my students. Not so. My exp
and judgment were on vacation. I was dealing with such
and frightening facts that, as I now realize, my attempts to di
my illness were somewhat erratic. I wanted my childre
understand with a minimum of effort on my part and so I prete
that they did.

I think it was good to attempt to demystify the word ca
by using it freely and sometimes capriciously until the chi
were bored by hearing it and it finally, as a word, lost muc
its impact. This came from a brainstorm when I was teac
sex education and had an anxious class say the words "p
and "vagina" until the giggling stopped and we could settle c
and learn some facts. In my own family I overlooked wl
knew about the concrete way children think and how vivid
imaginations are. Ben's assumption that cancer is contagious
very logical in terms of his experience and, because I knew b
as an adult, it was not even a part of my perception of the prok
I was hurt when he turned away from me, but attributed
his anger at my illness and a self-protective switch of prir
loyalty to his father in case I didn't make it. I was hurt by
rejection but very understanding. *What I did not do was conf*
him with this change in behavior. Thus we spent more th

year with limited hugging and when we did, I had a child who felt he was risking cancer just to have a snuggle with his mother.

I have learned that honesty in dealing with children and illness can indeed do much to dispel the "worst case scenario" that children so readily devise. The worst that a child can imagine is almost always an exaggerated horror.

I do not mean to recommend that we torture children with every detail and negative possibility when a parent is sick, but rather that we should not pretend that things are under control and not too serious when the child knows, as children can, that this is not true. The reality can be presented in a truthful but gentle way. After too many bungled attempts to soften the truth and protect each other, Ben has promised to ask the questions and I have promised to tell him the truth, even if it is bad news. Finally, we have built some trust and Ben can stop imagining horror shows. He knows now that it is better to ask me if he has a question or a worry and that I will be straight with him.

When Mom got cancer, I was almost ten years old. Now I am eleven and a lot more grown up. Then, I remember that I didn't seem very important in our family and almost all of the good things that happened while Mom was in the hospital happened away from home. Friends of the family and relatives were nice to me. Mom's school where she teaches sent me a beautiful, expensive little model car. I still keep it in the box so it won't get messed up. That first Christmas when Mom got home just in time to celebrate with us, she got more presents than anybody. I was glad she got them but Christmas is mostly for children and that year she got most of the attention.

I talked before about the way people treated me at school and a little about the way I acted. It wasn't too good. I've never been the kind of kid who sits still in school, but still I'm a pretty smart kid and get good grades in most of my subjects. I just work better standing up and moving around so I mess up on my report in things like "self-control" and "exhibits good study habits." My handwriting is very neat and I love math and reading. I like some of the things we do in school but I do like to do things my

own way. I am not perfect in school and probably haven't l
since I left first grade. Six years old was my best year ever.

    In fourth grade, after Mom got sick, things went wrong
me at school. My grades were still good but my behavior
really off the wall. A lot of the time I didn't even know I
disturbing the class and I got in trouble for dumb things
smearing powdered sugar on my face and making strange no
in class. I'd sneak in toys from home and fiddle with them.
and Mom and the guidance counselor all tried to talk to me
still I got bad notes almost every week. Mom made a barg
with me that if I could clean up my act in school, she would
me on a trip to Williamsburg, Virginia, a place we'd been be
and really loved. I blew it. Even with a treat like that, I
didn't behave right. The bad notes kept coming. I tried to bl
my trouble on the other kids and my teachers. I just couldn't
any way out. I decided I probably was a rotten kid.

PAT: Research tells us that traumatic change in a ten-
fourteen-year-old's life may cause attitude and behavior probl
which can affect the rest of his life. This age group is so vulnera
not having the shorter memory and less sophisticated thou
processes of a young child, but not being grown up enough
have begun the separation from the family and the str
self-involvement of adolescence which help protect older chilo
from the impact of the trouble on the home front. So M
experiences a guilt trip; all the nurturing and car pooling one
shouldered for years is now being obliterated by something
of your control, and "bad notes" appear with the regularity
half-eaten sandwich in the daily return of the lunch box.

    Ben, as he says, has always been an active learner, full of ic
and energy, able to learn best by standing at his desk contor
himself into strange postures as he cranks out his assignme
At home he spreads papers and debris in a ten-foot circle in fi
of the television. Despite this learning style, his work is excell
and his assignments complete. I have spent his entire school ca
hearing how bright, capable and "busy" he is. Under the bes

circumstances, Ben is fun, but he is a definite challenge in a conventional classroom.

In fourth grade, after my cancer was discovered, his less winning traits developed in inverse proportion to our inability to cope with them. His grades amazingly remained high but his behavior both at home and school became harder to live with. Mostly Ben made noise. He discovered whistling and practiced this new art constantly with ever increasing volume. Everything from "The Wedding March" to bird calls. If he discovered a theme he liked he'd repeat it for hours. When a problem came up that we would need to discuss with Ben, he would lose himself in his whistling, defying us to break through his concentration with mere words.

Often he and his dog Sam would go outside, anywhere away from all of us. From the house we could hear whistling from the barn, the woods, under a tree or encircling the house as Ben and Sam trudged around and around the circular driveway. We tried to live with this reasoning that it was his way of expressing something that desperately needed expression. He certainly knew that it got on the family's nerves and assured that he would eventually get our attention. I attempted to joke with him about it and told him that I was becoming known as "Whistler's Mother" within our circle of friends. I bought him the print which became a part of our permanent decor.

During this time, if Ben did something requiring a reprimand, he would immediately get angry and defensive with us. Everything that he did wrong was our fault. After all (according to Ben), dishes and dishwashers would not get broken if his unreasonable parents were more normal and would not insist that he help clean up the kitchen.

Things were not going smoothly and something needed to be done to get us back on track. I worried more about Ben's unhappiness than I did about his misbehavior. Certainly he brought home bad notes, but what concerned me more was his growing conviction that he was no longer the good kid that he had been in the lower grades. I was disturbed to learn that he considered first grade the apex of his life and that he was becoming more and more convinced that everything was downhill from that point.

We considered therapy for Ben or perhaps family therap᷉
all of us, but that would mean yet another car pool, the responsil᷉
of finding an appropriate counselor, and one more medical exp᷉
Also we were all exhausted, trying to cope with the overloa᷉
a day with too few hours.

We could have worked out a punishment system or a᷉
for behavior modification, both of which take energy, forti᷉
consistency, and imagination to carry out. We didn't have n᷉
of any of these qualities in reserve. This did leave the e᷉
option to wait things out and hope the problems would imp᷉
when the critical part of my treatment was complete.

On the plus side there was Sam, the dog who followed᷉
despite, or perhaps because of, the constant whistling.᷉
provided unquestioning and uncritical love and endured exce᷉
hugging mixed with stern orders issued by a confused and unha᷉
little boy. Sam was, and still is, Ben's best friend, someone᷉
loves him and doesn't talk back.

While Sam was indeed a godsend, and lessened our feelir᷉
guilt, we knew that something more was needed. After n᷉
thinking, I came up with an idea.

BEN: *I sometimes felt pretty lonely in my family while Mom was*
My oldest brother Jeb was away at college and, though he u᷉
or called sometimes, he was busy going to parties and stua᷉
and didn't have much time to think about what was goin᷉
here at home. My brother Sean was sixteen and though I k᷉
he worried about Mom, he didn't want to talk much, espec᷉
to me. We've always had some fights and picked on each o᷉
The year Mom was sick I think we got worse instead of be᷉

Sam, my dog, was my best friend during Mom's bad t᷉
He almost always came when I called him and he knew he c᷉
sleep on my bed even though it is against house rules. I c᷉
tell Sam anything and know he wouldn't tell anyone else or᷉
me I shouldn't say four letter words or have the nasty thou᷉
I sometimes had.

The other person I talked to was God. My family only᷉
to church for weddings and funerals, so I don't know too m᷉

about the God who lives in Church. Mom said that God is a spirit and it is in each of us as whatever we wish him to be. Or not at all, if that is the way we feel. Well, my God is kind of an old man because I really don't know what a spirit looks like. I think he is old because he has been around a long time. He is kind and, I think, a little fat. He is a sort of full time Santa Claus who cares for children but doesn't bring presents and all that stuff. His job is more important than that. He's the one who has control over everything.

I didn't tell Mom until we were writing about talking to God because I was afraid she would think it was silly. So he is my God and I'd make deals with him like I would work on my behavior if he'd let my mother get well. I slipped up sometimes on my end of the bargain, but Mom seems to be real healthy anyway. That's why I think God must be a very kind spirit or person. He is taking care of Mom and he understands I am just a kid and can mess up.

I was afraid that my mother would die. I knew she and Dad were afraid too. Sometimes I just wanted to run away or hide. When I couldn't I started whistling all the time to make noise and to shut out the horrible thoughts that were running around my brain. The sound of whistling fills my whole head. It helped when I didn't like the thoughts I was thinking to turn them off with noise. I didn't mean to drive my family crazy but I don't care that I did. After all, they were driving me crazy.

My problems at school were getting me down, as I really didn't want a reputation as a bad kid. I just didn't know how to stop. Half the time I didn't know what I was doing that was so awful and the other half I didn't care because I could make the other kids laugh and that made me feel like a regular kid again.

Then Mom came up with an idea.

"I Think I Can..."

One of the distressing aspects of a long illness, though perhaps less devastating than the reality of physical pain or the threat of death, is one's loss of control over happenings, both internal and external. From the moment my trouble was diagnosed, I became a patient. Though hospitals and medical personnel try to make the experience as endurable as possible, I felt I had entered a strange and frightening culture which uses new language and customs and in which I was very low on the organizational totem pole. Things were done to me, and although I signed the necessary forms, I was not in any shape to question or understand what the procedure or treatment involved.

In a hospital I became more childlike; meals became a high point of the day, they are delivered in mysterious little packages. I was cosseted, often called "Baby" or "Sweetie" by kind nurses; my schedule determined by the institution and, having great friends and family, they too joined in the game. When I was very sick we welcome this "take charge" atmosphere. Someone else would make me well.

In the beginning of my illness, I had many doctors and hospital staff to support me. In just a week I was turned out of the hospital to go home and cope as best I could with my remaining symptoms and fears.

Those of us determined to survive adopt a John Wayne bravado. We will make it despite the odds, despite the fact that our bodies feel they have been run over by a truck carrying fifty thousand pounds of bananas, and our battered souls are not too sure of the value of survival. Despite all this we will try to get well.

In a disease such as cancer with its often distressing treatn
bravado was not enough. It seemed to me and my family
life had become two steps forward and three steps back. M
of the treatment made me feel lousy and chipped away at
intention to be a "good soldier." Life had taken a new and
turn and was out of my control.

After the superactive phase of my cancer, diagnosis, surge
scans, extensive tests and examinations, I was left to
chemotherapy and try to fit it into an already shattered fa
routine. "Normality" no longer existed. It had to be redefi
Panic began to take hold.

I started devouring books about cancer and treatments. I
of other peoples' experiences and found that this helped alle
some of the sense of loneliness and isolation one feels as a
person in a healthy world.

About this time a friend introduced me to a book by O.
Simonton, Stephanie Matthews-Simonton, and James L. Creig
called *Getting Well Again*. The Simonton theory offered s
positive things I could actively *do* to help me feel better a
my situation. The authors basically feel that people respor
treatment and recover faster if they feel they have some co
of their physical responses and can learn to train their bodi
react in positive ways to the treatment they are receiving. Pat
can learn to take an active part in the way mind and body
messages back and forth from and to ourselves about reco
In short, we as patients regain control over some of our treat
and become active participants in our effort to recover rather
passive lumps upon which doctors do things.

Getting Well Again and the tapes adapted from it were a
help to me. The technique they describe involves several st
1. Relaxation
2. Affirmation
3. Visualization

Relaxation exercises acknowledge the relationship bet
excessive stress and illness and help the patient overcome
feeling of helpless panic that overwhelms us when we becom

Affirmation is a method by which we learn to believe in our body's ability to repair and make itself well again.

Visualization is a technique of using mental imagery to activate the body's defenses against disease by using symbols and images to allow the patient an active part in fighting his illness.

Many excellent books have been written on these topics and I have included a list of those I found helpful at the end of this book. I do believe that stress can exacerbate and even cause some illnesses. It is well documented that people who have had many or severe upheavals at some period in their lives are more likely to get sick within a six-month to two-year period after the stressful events. It seems to me that stress overload is inevitable for most children and adults at some time or another.

What I dislike about some of the literature on stress and its relationship to illness is that it implies that we are responsible for creating or poorly handling stress we encounter and this, in turn, makes us responsible for the illness we then "bring on ourselves." To make a sick person feel guilt because he is ill is counterproductive and cruel. It is nonsense.

I began the Simonton techniques shortly after my return from the hospital and found, after practice, that they calmed me and restored some confidence in my ability to hang on and get well. Bill gave me a beautiful crystal that I let hang in the sunlight from my window. Staring at the shifting rainbows of color began for me the process of "letting go." As my anxiety would fade, I'd shut my eyes and try to catch the colors from the crystal in my mind. Listening to the tape while doing this helped me further relax and I would find myself in a pleasant state somewhere between waking and sleeping. *Getting Well Again* suggests visualizing a beautiful place in nature that makes you feel at peace. This worked for me also.

After I was relaxed, by the Simonton method, I started imagining the weak cancer cells being attacked by my ever strengthening immune system. The white cells would increase in strength and number to destroy the confused cancer cells. Because I had a severe case of anemia I visualized the red cells multiplying and making the body well and strong. How these things are visualized

is a matter of individual creativity and can become quite elab
and enjoyable.

Good self-help techniques reinforce conventional me
treatment rather than replace it. Thus I pictured the drugs
in chemotherapy as strong ammunition entering my body
blowing up any cancer cells in its path. I am sure this image
embedded in my subconscious after years of living with small
playing war throughout my house and garden. I would a
that the "ammunition" was strong and would sometimes l
innocent cells causing nausea, fatigue and other side effects.
pain I used my spectrum of color and bright light to bath
area where things hurt, and this brought relief. Finally I w
tell myself over and over how I was getting well, how str
was feeling, how the cancer was gone from my body. Repet
a form of self-hypnosis, while I relaxed helped affirm my reco
I'd play tapes repeating the same message as I'd drift off to s

There are many ways to approach this taking part in reco
individually, in groups, prayer, and formal therapy. I believe
approach works because we become participants in our f
rather than helpless victims.

I began my "therapy" alone as I live in a rural place
didn't have the energy to seek out or drive to a group. My fa
soon learned to respect Mom's meditating and to leave me a
when they heard the frequent drone of one of
relaxation/visualization tapes. We all saw that some very po
results were evolving from this process and everybody was
to see me find some resource, some way to cope with the terri
things that had happened to me.

BEN: *It wasn't too long after Mom came home from the hospital*
she started listening to those tapes. My mom never does any
a little bit so the tapes and meditation went on a lot of the
The family learned that when we heard this voice going on
on that it was best to leave Mom alone.

Sometimes I would sneak in and, if I was quiet, she w
let me stay. I heard this guy on the tape telling her how
cancer cells are and that she could kill them herself becaus

body has strong fighter cells. Mom really started to believe this stuff and she read every book she could find about it. She thinks that the more you know, the bigger the chance you might find something that works for you. I didn't mind Mom and her tapes; I was all for anything that would help her and make her better. It did sound funny though, this tape saying the same thing over and over. It also meant still more time when Mom was busy with something and I had to go away.

One day Mom called me into her room especially to talk. I knew she'd been really worried about my bad notes and the way I'd been acting. I just kind of stuck around at home; I didn't call my friends much. I didn't really like anybody much. Anyway Mom told me why she did the tapes and said she thought maybe I could do it with her. She said that meditation wasn't just tapes and wasn't just for sick people. She said it mostly is a way to relax and feel better about yourself. To tell the truth I didn't think much of the idea, but we all tried hard to go along with Mom then, so I let her talk. Plus she said we could do it together and I would be helping her. So even if it is silly, I'd get to be with Mom and, as I said before, I couldn't think of anything better to change the way I'd been feeling, so why not give it a shot?

The first time Mom and I tried meditation, it was pretty funny. We sat cross-legged on the bed and held hands. We didn't use a tape. Instead Mom talked in this soft sleepy voice about feeling your toes relax and tingle, then your ankles. She was ready to do my whole body piece by piece. I started to giggle; the whole scene seemed pretty dumb to me. She didn't get mad or anything. She just said that it did look a little silly. She asked me if I'd try some stuff anyway so I did.

She asked me to tense some muscles in my face and hold them that way. Then she'd say to let it go. I could really feel a difference. After we did that for a while she had me draw a picture in my mind of a happy peaceful place. That was easy for me. I saw a field of waving wheat as a gentle breeze goes through it. I am sitting on the edge of a small pond and there is a frog for company. The only sound is the swoosh of the wind through the grass,

water sounds, and a little croak from the frog. It was a
place to be and I felt as though I was sharing it with her.

Finally she asked me to send her some of the positive e
from myself to her. She said I could send it through my h
to her and she would send some back to me. I couldn't be
it at first but then I actually felt something in me flowing
Mom and tingles of energy from her going into my hands. It
weird but good and I began to think there might be some
to this stuff.

After I got used to the idea Mom and I meditated pretty c
I even borrowed one of her tapes which helped you like yo
better by picturing someone you hate and then forgiving t
On that tape, the lady said that you didn't have to stay au
so I'd play it at bedtime and fall asleep while she was still tal

Meanwhile Mom and I tried lots of different ways to med
which were fun and kept it from getting boring. She u
sometimes light a candle and we would stare at it and the
to see the flame with our eyes closed. Mom would tell me t
to see the flame in the center of my forehead and make
bright and steady as I could. I went along with it but I'm
sure what that was supposed to do.

Another thing Mom taught me was to pick a word or ph
and just say it either in your head or out loud over and ov
you don't think any other thoughts. I picked "Sam," my
name, and said it inside my brain. It worked kind of like whis
did, only quieter.

The best thing Mom came up with was picturing wha
wanted to happen. Mom would talk softly about school and
classroom and I would try to see what she was talking abo
my head. She would say, "See Ben sitting quietly at his
He is feeling peaceful and good about himself. He doesn't
to distract anyone. He is sitting quietly listening to wha
teacher is saying. See the teacher who is smiling at Ben bec
he has done his work and is listening. Ben is feeling good a
being in school; he does not need to make crazy noises. B
calm; Ben feels good about his life."

As you can see, Mom repeated this stuff over and over. The funny thing, though, is that it did seem to work. It would come back at school and I would feel good like I had with Mom and the day would work out. Maybe she hypnotized me. I don't know. It did make life easier.

One time when we were both sick of meditating about school, Mom asked me if there was anything else I'd like to change or work on. I said that I hadn't had a hit in baseball all season and I'd like to change that. We did our relaxation and then she talked about feeling the bat in my hand and feeling power in my body and arms. She had me picture myself at home plate even down to the blue sky and all the kids in the field. I saw myself waiting for the pitch. At exactly the right moment I would swing the bat and feel the ball connect with the wood and go sailing. Both Mom and I could actually feel the power of the hit I would make.

That night, at baseball, I got my first hit of the season. This stuff can really work.

Ten Good Things

People need to feel some measure of control over things that happen to them. Although helpless to prevent some of the trauma fate hands us, we do have some power of choice as to how we respond—how we shape our lives after unavoidable changes occur.

This consciousness of choice is important for children, especially those in the ten to fourteen age group who are old enough to recognize their dependency and who are just entering that stage of development where they are anxious to take control of some parts of their lives.

Ben, like most children his age, wants a say in the way his life is managed. This is putting it mildly; he is entering that charming period where he questions most decisions made by his parents and gives us the clear impression that he is totally unsure of our competence both as parents and as reasoning human beings. He pushes us away and feels rejected when we go. Being eleven is not an easy row to hoe.

Like most children Ben apparently had a picture of life as he thought it should be. To have this image shattered by a sudden blow forced him through the looking glass into a country where all the road signs seemed to be written in a foreign language.

Relaxation and meditation exercises began the process of rediscovering ourselves and stilling the panic. After the initial awkwardness of sitting quietly, a feat in itself for Ben, and dealing with the embarrassment of a new and strange experience, our time together became something we both looked forward to. It was important to allow silliness if that was the initial response. It didn't hurt me to let up a little and act light-hearted too. The

object of the meditation and relaxation was to make us both
better, and if a good laugh could help accomplish that goa
the better. The important thing was that we both regain a s
of control. This is not a teacher-to-pupil exercise, but a
where two people can share something and achieve a r
comfortable feeling about life and its happenings. So, if eith
us became temporarily frivolous, we had the rare reward
shared moment of pleasure.

When Ben began to enjoy our sessions, we branched out
tried many different ways of relaxing and visualizing. Our
was very basic: we wanted positive time together. It was a
when we could relate person to person rather than as adu
kid. I truly needed help from him and the times we sat toge
with our hands touching were the most meaningful for me c
the exercises we attempted. We actually could feel the flov
energy and support flowing between us, like mild electrical chat
Ben was giving something to me; I was having the reinforcer
of his presence to help me to continue the program I had se
myself.

After our set routine of relaxation exercises and q
meditation, we found that trying a variety of approaches kept
sessions fresh. To explore the possibilities of these techniqu
fun. The sky's the limit. We could try for any desired outc
through visualization. It made us both feel, if not omnipo
at least more in control of things. It also taught us both
visualization is not solely a "sick to well" exercise but rath
means to improve the quality of our lives even in ordinary ti

Ben has always expressed his feelings about life in a fa
dramatic way. It was comforting to me to believe that he
getting it all out with his outbursts and temperamental spells
took a long time for me to accept that he was expressing se
emotional pain and not just "going through a stage." Wh
was experiencing such personal pain, I minimized his unhappir
This is self-protective but also indicative of the way we
grown-ups, expect children to cope. Because they are young,
try to believe that their problems are less profound. We w
them to "go out and play," and that will take care of their troul

We encourage them to participate in sports which do provide an excellent physical outlet for tension. However, it seems to me, as a teacher and parent, that children are expected to sit for fairly long periods of time with a figure of authority making sure that they do. No matter what is going on in their personal lives, a child is expected to "be good." A "good kid" is usually defined within a school setting as one who sits quietly, does the assignment without asking too many questions and generally does not make waves. I wonder how many adults could survive the limits and expectations put on a child in the course of an average school week, not counting the added difficulty of unusual stress. A child is usually expected to sit an hour or more and do homework when he gets home. I know that I could not possibly perform as well, and certainly not as quietly, as children are expected to do. It must be especially difficult when your position in the organization doesn't leave you much leeway for complaint.

As Ben learned to visualize, his behavior and attitude toward school dramatically improved and he began to develop new ways to adapt his new control to his school day. I let him in on a very secret technique handed down to me by a wise and wonderful teacher, Ann Gilpin. It can only be used with great discretion and I feel a twinge of guilt in revealing the secret here. As it can only be effectively used by a student who has mastered visualization, perhaps I am not putting too many teachers at risk. I think I'll let Ben tell it; that way I am not directly responsible for the consequences.

What Mom is hinting at is a wonderful way to get back at a teacher who is driving you nuts. I guess it could be worked on the people at home too, but I haven't tried it yet.

What you do is sit very still at your desk in school and stare at the teacher and concentrate on him or her as though you are listening to every word he or she is saying. Then, when you feel the power in you, you focus on a part of the teacher's body. I usually try for the bottom, and I try to make that part of the teacher itch. I can do it by visualizing and by sending messages to the body part. Itch . . . itch . . . itch.

It worked; the teacher scratched just where I sent the thor
and I didn't get in trouble as I was just sitting there. The tea
thought I was being better than usual. Little did he know
think it must be part of some old voodoo ritual or somethin
do know that Mrs. Gilpin told Mom about it so I'd have a
to keep from ending up in the principal's office.

I guess if a person feels really angry or mean, he could men
stick pins in people, but I haven't had to do that so far.

Things did get better for me at school after Mom and I
meditation. I don't mean to say everything was perfect or
I suddenly loved school. Sometimes I got sick of meditating
didn't want to bother with it. Still I am glad I learned how
if things ever get real tough for me again, I would probabl
back to it.

Maybe it was the meditation or maybe I started to get
to what had happened to Mom, but life got easier around
house toward the end of Mom's chemotherapy. She starte
come to my baseball games and she would yell like the res
the parents. We seemed to have time to laugh again. I'm
sure any of us really believed that she would ever get off t
anticancer drugs, but she was counting the days and trying
hard not only to keep going, but to put some fun back in
life. She was excited about her new garden and I liked b
with her when she would go on and on about flower names.
would weed and prune and I could help. It really made me ha
to see her want to do something besides lie around and be s

Mom started walking more then too and making an effor
get stronger. She seemed to have hope again, maybe from
own meditation time, and that made the rest of the family
like we were going to make it. We were all tired of having a
mother and, even though we knew she couldn't help it, w
least wanted the chemotherapy to end so she would be more
her old self.

PAT: Battling through chemotherapy was miserable but there v
brief times when the nausea and exhaustion would lift and
living became in those moments a glorious gift. My garden

most special. A present from a friend, it had seeds from Monet's garden in France. We planted them by color and size having no idea what would appear. Once the seeds sprouted we had the fun of trying to identify them and finding new surprises daily coming into bloom. This unpredictable garden helped me to generate energy to weed and plant, and I'd lose myself in the sunlight and simplicity of physical work. The strength I'd always taken for granted was now a rare experience and one I treasured.

I tried, encouraged by my family and visualization, to become stronger both in body and spirit. I began to take walks and wander along familiar paths through the woods. In my journal I listed the small joys and victories that made it possible for me to keep trying. This was an activity I'd come up with when I would feel so low I'd want to give up, give in, literally lie down and die. I'd force myself to list "ten good things" for the day. At times this became a monumental task, as I could see nothing worth surviving for. Still, once I'd try, a list would grow. One list included:

- A hug from Ben when he woke up
- Visiting the first crocus even though it was raining
- Long fingernails: they kept growing in spite of everything
- Buying groceries and feeling well enough to plan a whole week's meals
- Potato chips
- Chloe, my cat, coming in and sleeping on my stomach
- Thinking about shrimp for Saturday night supper
- Friends calling and caring about me
- A hematocrit of 35, only one point below where it was when I first went into the hospital
- A chocolate rose in my mailbox from my secret friend
- Touching toes with Bill at night so I could go to sleep and not feel all alone.

I began to believe I could make it, as the chemotherapy
to come was measured in weeks rather than months.

One special day I remember leaving the house with the
Sam and walking down the farm road with nothing but trees
fields. Ben came and joined us on his bike. Bright blue sky
the first warm sun of spring. No other living creatures b
mourning dove and the dog leaping and blending with the
tan stubble of the winter fields. Ben and I hugged and
horrendous winter was for the moment forgotten. We che
wild chives and ran through the field breathing dragon-like drea
onion on each other. We laughed and rested together on the
grass as Sam raced crazily about, glad to be away and outs
The sun shone on us all.

The ordinary is extraordinary.

Picking Up The Pieces

Chemotherapy finally ended in June, six months after the whole nasty illness had been discovered. As Ben said in his section, I am not one to do things in moderation, so I immediately set up an appointment with a reconstructive surgeon to discuss my options and to make some decisions about the next step I would take. Because I planned to return to full time teaching in the fall, I felt that the only time I could plan reconstructive surgery was during the summer vacation. This allowed very little time for me to rest and recover from the effects of chemotherapy before plunging into the next ride on the medical merry-go-round. The surgery I chose is relatively new and involves using part of the abdominal muscle and repositioning it to form a breast without an artificial implant of any kind.

The operation is an exciting procedure; it is amazing to think that a surgeon can rearrange one's body using what is already there and end up with a patient who, with minor scarring, is able to navigate life looking and feeling whole without the problems of silicone. The "breast" is living tissue; it loses or gains weight along with the rest of the body. It doesn't have the sensitivity and feeling of the original, but it does feel real. An added bonus of this method of reconstruction is that it involves a "tummy tuck," which means that one loses the extra belly some of us acquire over the years. What a morale boost to regain a flat stomach and feel that the excess has gone in a good cause.

The disadvantage to this method of reconstruction is that the initial surgery is long and arduous and one must stay in the hospital for five days. The recovery period is fairly long and uncomfortable

as both the chest and abdominal area are involved. I went
six months of relative inactivity while on the chemotherapy
six weeks of training to get in shape for the surgery, which
scheduled for mid-summer. So singleminded was I that Bill
I didn't allow ourselves even a weekend away. Vacation
wasn't in the picture.

Friends have often joked about how I Christmas shop mo
ahead. In school I was the rare student who did an assi
paper right away to get it over with. I would then use the
saved to least advantage by partying or simply doing nothin
think I had a bit of that spirit left as I wanted the last mise
year to be part of the past as quickly as possible. Medita
notwithstanding, I retained some of my native impatience in war
things completed.

The boys' vacations did work out. Jeb went away to v
as a camp counselor, and Sean spent two sessions in lacrosse ca
Ben was enrolled in his first sleepover camp and seemed ple
at the prospect. My husband Bill, in desperation, bought hir
a canoe so he could find temporary escape on the lake near
house.

I was definitely on a roll. I carried a folder I put tog
and titled "Mostly Medical" around with me and tried to orga
and manage this new stage of my treatment. I spent six w
prior to surgery having cardiology studies to make sure that
heart was strong enough for the upcoming operation and dona
blood for autologous transfusions. In this procedure, the pa
donates blood to be used during surgery. The obvious advan
to this method is that one receives one's own blood, which ass
compatible transfusion and eliminates the possibility of contra
blood-transmitted diseases. I did everything I could think
try to make sure the surgery would go smoothly and success
This time I was not in shock; I tried to prepare, educate my
and make my own decisions. I wanted to feel some control
time.

I became a kind of human dynamo. This was part of
reaction to the end of chemotherapy. I had done a m
countdown to the date when it would be over and looked at

day as a milestone, the turning point from sick to well. As it came nearer the family began to hope that some of their extra duties would also let up. Bill informed me, even before my last treatment, that I could start picking up my own milk on the way home from work! Everybody was tired of taking care of me and wanted me to do my part again.

The pressure mounted further when my school offered me a promotion. I was asked to help set up and head a new middle school branch to open in September, just five weeks after my surgery. This was such an affirmation of survival and of people's belief in me that I never considered turning it down.

Summer is supposed to be a time when you don't work very hard. I remember when I was a little kid I made up a song that went, "In the summer, I can QUIT!" Short song, but I sang it over and over and didn't do anything for as long as I could get away with it. No more homework, no regular bedtime, no early getting up, late suppers on the screened porch. Summer is tubing in the river, fishing and lying in a hammock; it is crayfish. And swimming in a friend's pool.

Usually I clean my room in the summer. I mean REALLY clean it and throw out all the clothes and toys and schoolwork I don't need anymore. Most every summer I grow a lot too because Mom always has to get rid of last year's school clothes and never can figure out just when they got too small. We've gone to California, Williamsburg and Busch Gardens, but we usually go to the ocean.

That summer I was going to camp. I'd never been to sleepover camp before and I was pretty excited about it. Sean, my brother, had been to this camp before and told me about the cabins right on the edge of Chesapeake Bay. He told me about a carnival they have at the camp that has a kissing booth and how the camp has a ghost who lives in an abandoned cabin in the woods. This was going to be my first time away from home and I was really ready to get out of there.

Mom was just finishing up her chemotherapy treatments around then and kept telling us how much better she would be when she

stopped. Well, she finally stopped, but I couldn't see that
was any different. She was still very tired and her hair, w
she didn't have much of, began growing in about five diffe
colors. She kept trying to push herself to be well, but she
wasn't. The more she would push, the crankier she got and w
take a lot of it out on the rest of the family. She was har
live with then being so impatient with herself. She just mad
rest of us tired and impatient with her too.

Mom would decide to do some big job like scrub the p
or wash the dog. She'd start in and then get too tired to fi
She'd talk to my brother and me in this incredibly mean i
and tell us to do it. She made it sound like it was our fault,
everything was our fault. I didn't even care if the porch was
clean. It seemed like most of the time she was mad at all i
and none of us could do anything right. There was just no plea
her.

I couldn't wait to get to camp.

PAT: It is so frustrating to reach a longed-for goal like comple
chemotherapy and find no appreciable difference in the da
day routine. I guess I expected the side effects and emoti
exhaustion to lift magically as I recovered from my last shot
swallowed my last pill. There was a high to having comp.
something difficult and our friends and family celebrated
"coming out." Mostly I was still reeling through this period
needed much support. So was the family. They too had
staggering toward the finish line and hoping for big change
summer approached with promises of no schoolwork and a mc
"back to her old self."

What energy I had left after arranging my summer me
agenda went into all those household chores I had put off du
chemo. As if to prove to myself and everybody around me
I truly had recovered, I began a mission to put our house
lives into order. Fortunately we had a wonderful cleaning wo
who had helped keep the house from collapsing under dirt du
my treatments. She was so much better at cleaning than I t
gratefully left that area to her. Now she was planning to re

to a full-time job just as I was noticing all the things we'd left undone in the last six months. There was the nightmare in the attic where we'd thrown everything we couldn't find a place for downstairs. The dog had left offerings of fur in every room. I don't think anyone had brushed him for a year. The screened porch had been taken over by spiders and cats who, like the dog, had left their souvenirs.

I would wake up with an illusion of energy and throw myself into some project, determined to accomplish it, and then run out of steam in the middle of it. I would whine at the kids to finish whatever it was. In my frustration and anger at being so weak, I'd blame them and do my best to make them as miserable as I was.

At first they would step in fairly cheerfully to bail me out, but the degree of sullenness increased as the summer progressed. They seemed to spend long periods of time on the phone arranging to be absent from home.

I wondered later why we didn't all go away as we had in the past, but I understand now our reluctance to be together with less space or fewer escape hatches. We had all asked extraordinary things from one another. We had given to each other all we had to give. We needed separate time.

I knew that Mom had to go back to the hospital for more surgery that summer, but this time she explained exactly what they were going to do to her. She showed me drawings of the operation, and even though it was a little gory, I did feel better about knowing what was going to happen to her. She explained that this was not an operation to get rid of cancer. I'm glad she said that, as I kind of thought that most operations were because of cancer. In my life so far, they all had been. This operation was to build a breast, not a real one, but one made out of part of her stomach, which was a little too fat anyway. When the doctor finished, her body would have balance and her two sides would match. This operation made sense to me and I wasn't as afraid as I had been before. I even went with her to the hospital for her tests before the surgery. I remember going to the blood lab and watching

while the technician put a big needle in her arm to take (
pint of blood to save for her operation. It didn't bother n
watch her get stuck and I didn't feel weird when I saw the l
coming out. I decided I probably should become a veterin
when I grow up. It was interesting. The only bad thing
that Mom got juice and cookies when it was over and I d
That didn't seem right to me.

A couple of weeks before Mom was to go into the hos,
we got me ready for camp. It was fun collecting things: flash
bug repellent, little tube of toothpaste, powder, soap in a st
box you could close. We put my name on all my clothes,
on my pillow. Mom thought I'd lose everything, I guess. Fi
the big day came and Mom and I drove over the Chesapeake
Bridge to the camp. We stopped for lunch on the way d
and I remember staying in the bathroom a long time. I bego
realize I was really going away and my stomach was feeli
little nervous. Still I wanted to go; I couldn't wait to get a
from home.

Camp looked great when I first saw it. It had screened co
along the bay just like Sean said. It had a big dining hall
picnic tables and a porch with rockers where kids and couns
could sit and talk. There was a pool, canoes and fields for go
There was a camp store where you could buy tee shirts, c
and soda. Mom and I unloaded my stuff in my cabin and I
my counselor. I was anxious for Mom to leave and so she

The best thing that happened during that week at camp
when lightning hit the flagpole and it split in two and fell
The rest of the time the kids in my cabin ganged up and
really mean to me. Most of them had been there before
thought they owned the place. There was one other new kid
was left out too. Now I wish I'd tried to get to know him bec
he was nice, but I didn't try then. I'm sorry I didn't now.

One night I got into a fight with one of these kids who
my comb and threw it in the mud. That was the last stra;
ran away from camp and stayed in a ditch all through di
Finally one of the counselors found me crying and crying.
was nice; he said those kids really were mean and that I sh

just stay away from them. That turned out to be pretty easy, as I topped off the week by getting sick with a fever of 103 degrees and spent two days in the infirmary. Part of the time passed there and I didn't even know it. I do know I got free popsicles there. At least the nurse was nice.

I was so glad to see Mom. She was unhappy that I had hated camp. She had wanted me to get away from it all and have some fun. No deal.

It was such a relief to me that Ben was getting away from home for a little while and going to such a fun place. He, more than any of us, was so vulnerable and had been hurt badly by the events of the past year.

Camp was to be an escape; a chance for Ben to be with kids doing things kids enjoy. He'd get away from the stress at home and a chance to break away from his position as baby of the family. Sean had loved this camp; it had really helped him grow up. I wanted the same for Ben.

We didn't hear from Ben while he was gone, which we took as a positive sign that he was too busy enjoying himself to write letters. When I arrived at the end of the week and found a shaken, unhappy child, my heart ached for him. We did a lot of hugging and reassuring that he wouldn't ever have to go back. We packed the car in record time and beat feet out of there.

Looking back, I wonder if Ben would have been happy in any camp that summer. He had been under a lot of pressure also and had shown signs of depression at home, not wanting to call his friends or do much away from me or the house. He just didn't have the energy that summer to crack a closed group of kids. Add strep throat to that scenario and it was total misery.

Despite the harassment we dish out to one another within the family, we did understand the pain that each of us was experiencing. Even though we all bitched at regular intervals, we also provided a safety net for one another. We weren't ready to walk the wire without it.

Ben and I went home.

Home Free?

After camp, home didn't look so bad. Besides, in less than a week Mom was going into the hospital and I was going to my Aunt Lee's house, where I was pretty sure they would be nice to me. I don't know why I hated that camp so much; I just know that I would never ever go back. Looking back, there were things that I like about the idea of camping. Being with a bunch of kids, sleeping in a cabin, getting to swim every day. Maybe I'll try another one next summer.

When Mom went in for her operation, my aunt picked me up and took me down to her house. She and my cousins live near the water so I could go crabbing and fishing. Their house is in a regular neighborhood with lots of kids so I could go out and play anytime I wanted to without carpooling. I love living in the country, but having kids around any time you want to play is neat. Also, I was the only boy in the house and I got to tease my girl cousins. I think it was a change for my aunt to have a boy around. I got to go to an Orioles baseball game and spend money. It was a great week. I knew Mom was all right, so I just enjoyed myself. Actually I forgot all about her for awhile.

When I came back home, Mom had just come home too. She was upstairs again in her room. This time she had even more bandages all over. She had staples which the doctor used along with stitches to hold things together. Gross. She couldn't stand up straight and she spent most of her time back in bed. In a funny way that seemed kind of normal to me. I guess we had gotten used to her being sick. Really I couldn't remember too well what Mom had been like before she got cancer.

Anyway, she wasn't as sick as she had been on chemother
she was just tired and stiff and uncomfortable. It was pig
that summer, so I spent a lot of time with her in the air-conditio
bedroom. That was kind of fun; we watched television toge
and friends came by to visit and bring us cakes. On hot n
I'd bring in my sleeping bag and camp out on the floor. I c
keep her company and be cool at the same time.

PAT: Returning to the hospital could have been a horror show,
was bound to bring back memories of my previous visits. Know
this, I tried to use my meditation as much as possible to ease
apprehension. Actually, the preliminaries to my admission w
kind of fun. The staff at the hospital was obviously glad to I
a well patient coming in for a procedure, which was no
emergency and was intended to restore rather than rem
something. Everyone there knew Dr. McGibbon, my pl;
surgeon, and had a success story involving a "body by McGibb
I began to get excited as the reality of what I planned to do
in. The atmosphere at the hospital was so cheerful that I
Ben along on one of my pre-op visits and he too caught
enthusiastic outlook about the surgery. This time, as Ben
there was time for us to discuss and explain what was goin;
happen, even drawings to illustrate the operation. A little
graphic, I avoided studying them too closely, but for Ben, I t
they were a comfort. Children have stronger stomachs for o
people's ordeals.

So Ben took off for my sister's loaded down with crab
and fishing gear. He was extremely busy all week, and accor
to both Ben and Lee, didn't give me a thought. And so, fin
Ben got a break.

The same optimistic feelings went with us as Bill and I che
me into the hospital for the actual surgery. Here was a pat
the doctors could "fix" and make much happier in the proc
My pre-op training proved invaluable. Before the operating r
sent the gurney for me, I did some stretching exercises, gues
rightly that this might be the last free movement I'd get for c
a while. I had practiced this experience, visualizing myself b

wheeled into surgery feeling calm and confident. As I waited on the cart, I did some escape meditation. I think I was off in the moors of Scotland when I was put out by the anesthesiologist.

I can't minimize the miserable first twenty-four hours following surgery. I woke up in pain with drains and tubes all over. I tried meditation; I tried to recapture my excitement about my new body. No dice. I couldn't move at all and everything hurt. The pain shots were wonderful; oblivion was the best place to be for those initial hours.

After the first phase of recovery passed, I improved rapidly and gradually was able to substitute some of the pain killing drugs with mind control. Dr. McGibbon urged me not to be a heroine, so I looked forward to those jabs in the bottom for as long as I needed them. Self-help doesn't mean martyrdom. Within two days I was up, sort of, and beginning the hospital shuffle down the hall. Bit by bit I regained strength, and after five days I went home, stapled and sore, to continue my metamorphosis.

My newly air-conditioned bedroom was a haven from the hot humid Maryland summer. It was filled with flowers, pretty nightgowns, friends stopping by with goodies and staying to have a celebration drink with us. And Ben on the floor, keeping watch, keeping me company. Things were definitely looking up.

I remember that time as marvelously superficial. It was a time of glossy magazines. I don't think I had a serious thought for a month. I enjoyed my new body, slipping into pretty new nightgowns and sundresses without worrying about the prosthesis or the need to wear a bra. It was not a time for introspection. Rather it was a time to feel good, having survived and been brave through the surgery. I was beginning to believe in the completion of a nasty period of my life. Ten pounds had dropped off and my stomach was flat. Hot damn. My hair continued to grow albeit silver and straight. I began to think of things I hadn't been able to consider for months. Sean's Latin grades and how to help him, redecorating musty areas of the house. I felt like I was coming back from a long trip. I even began to read, which seemed a sign to me that I was at last coming down from the experience.

Part of me still wondered if they had done biopsies during operation, but I figured they would tell me if anything was wr I put that possibility on a back burner as I really didn't wan think about the past. I did my anti-stress tapes to try to ha the healing and get all my innards working again. My big problem was falling asleep. I was so wired for survival th couldn't let go enough to allow myself a solid night's rest. doctor prescribed a mild sedative and, feeling a bit of a fa for being unable to use my mental exercises to treat the insom I took them. I rationalized that this is the legitimate use for t drugs and it was better to get the rest than to send myself (guilt trip because I couldn't sleep. I must add that I did become dependent on the pills, and I am grateful that I had alternative to spending large parts of the night awake uncomfortable. It was a relief to be a little easy on myself.

BEN: *As the days passed Mom got stronger and stronger. She over*
it like Mom does and tried to can tomatoes two weeks after
got home. Then she'd get mad again at everybody and burst
tears. She couldn't drive so I was stuck at home unless some
could pick me up. It got pretty boring and I watched a lo
television. I kept waiting for an end to bad things and wonde
if there ever would be one. Mom kind of disappeared into he
doing her nails and dying her hair. She was starting to feel be
and was a little selfish about it. Life for me was pretty bor
but when I'd tell Mom she'd just say that at least I'd gotte
vacation and she hadn't. That was true but by the end of
summer a kid really can run out of things to do.
About four weeks after the operation Mom went into a
stage. Suddenly she had all these ideas for fixing up our ho
She asked me what I wanted most of all to do and I told her
new room." Whammo! She decided to change everybody's roc
around. My brother Sean would move to Jeb's big room on
third floor, I would move to Sean's room which is bigger t
mine, and Jeb, who is almost always away at college, would
my old little room. Mom went into all this like she had all
energy in the world. I remember going to the store and buy

furniture and a rug and other stuff for the changed rooms. Mom made everybody clean out all their drawers and desks and boxes. That was horrible. I didn't know I had so much stuff. We would all get tired of rearranging and Dad and Jeb would ask us what the big rush was. But once Mom starts something, watch out! Finally we did get moved though it took a lot of arguing and was not much fun. For a while I didn't really like my new room. Sure it was bigger and all cleaned up, but I felt I was in somebody else's place and I missed my little room. I didn't say too much about this to Mom or she would have gotten very mad. I'd just sneak back into my old room some nights after Jeb had gone back to college. I felt safe there and I wasn't sure I liked my grown-up room. I don't do that anymore; I've gotten used to the change.

I never will forget how strong Mom was when she set her mind to something. Phew. A person has to be careful about telling my mother that they're bored and have nothing to do.

In the weeks following the surgery, I got stronger and stronger. Naturally I had to test this new strength and, as is often my problem, I overdid it. There were so many things I suddenly wanted to accomplish. There was my neglected garden. There was a vegetable patch chock full of tomatoes, squash and peppers screaming to be preserved. Ben described the "great room switch" which took incredible energy and managed to offend everybody in the house before it was accomplished.

I've never, before or since, felt such vitality. Hyperactive would probably be a better word, but I didn't realize it at that time. At the end of the day I'd have attacks of rapid heartbeat but I had had a recent cardiac work-up and had been pronounced fit. I put it down to excitement over recovery and overdoing a little bit.

When I finished playing Superwoman at home, I tackled my new job of starting up the middle school. Recruiting my boys to do the heavy work, I organized classrooms and the office, figured out a schedule, and amassed and arranged books and materials. The other teachers and I bought equipment, decided rules and,

miraculously, opened on the first day looking remarkably li]
going operation.   Teaching and administrating was exhaus
and exhilarating. I was well at last.

At home I began to take over my former roles and trie(
relieve my husband of some of the cooking, shopping and enc
details he had shouldered during the last year. I felt so good w
he came home at night to a well cooked meal that he had no
in providing. People had given so much to me during my illr
That hadn't been easy for me as I am much better at being str
The long period of being unable to do things for myself and
family was not natural.

I felt that I had been endowed with some new energy
that sleep, rest and reflection were no longer necessary for
survival. I was on an energy high. Then out of the blue, my
was rear-ended, causing extensive damage. A dear friend of r
had a recurrence of her breast cancer. My boss, the head of
school, became ill, leaving me little back-up in my new posit
My house of cards began to collapse.

B E N :   *School started as it always does right after Labor Day. By*
my room looked terrific, as I had put up some posters and arrar
my desk just right for the beginning of the year. Mom and I u
shopping for school supplies and she let me get everything I nee
from folders to pens to dividers. It is really fun to shop for sc
supplies; everything is fresh and clean and you haven't messe(
even one piece of notebook paper. It is fun to organize it all
get everything exactly as you want it for the first day. Mom
me a new backpack for my books and an insulated lunch [
that I could also use on camping trips. She bought me a bu
of new clothes and was much better than she used to be a
spending money. Getting ready for school is a little like Christ
You look forward to using all new things and wearing new clo
and seeing your friends again.

I began the fifth grade that year, the last year in elemen
school. It was okay but the principal had changed the kids arc
and most of my best friends were in another class. It was
to be the oldest class in the school though, and I was given

job of putting the kindergarten kids on the bus so they wouldn't get lost. I liked that.

I also had signed up for band that year, and we rented a baritone, which I learned to play. A baritone is a big brass instrument like a small tuba, and it makes a big noise. I could drive Sean bananas with it and he couldn't do anything because I was practicing.

Mom was doing great by now. She went to her job every day and did the shopping and cooked dinner. I started to remember what normal life was like and began to realize that she was getting well. She even signed me up for soccer on weeknights and Saturdays. She came to most of the games and got very excited about our team. It was a great team. I got the position of goalie and was pretty good. I didn't care if I did get kicked in the head as long as I could keep that ball out of the goal. I made some good saves that season. Mom would get a little worried that my teeth might get kicked in, but I didn't even care. Our team won the championship for our age group and league that year. I had never been on a winning team ever, not in any sport. We fought hard for that championship and it sure felt great when we made it.

Fall was good that year. Things at home and school had settled down, and I don't think I worried about Mom too much. It was funny, she would get very tired and when the family would snuggle down to watch "The Cosby Show" and "Family Ties," she'd miss most of it by falling asleep. Then she'd wake up and complain that she couldn't get a good night's sleep. Most of the time, though, she cooked dinner and kept the house going.

We'd started planning for Halloween and looking forward to the holidays. Then, sometime in October, some jerk hit her car. She wasn't hurt, but she began to fall apart after that. I don't think she was as strong as we had thought.

Crash Landing

In a way the car accident was a catalyst, exposing the sham of my super energy. I was innocently waiting to make a left turn when suddenly my entire body was jolted and my car decreased its length by four inches from the impact. There was no warning; the driver behind me just came on too fast and forgot to use her brakes. The odds of this happening sometime, after twenty years of accident-free driving, were against me. These things happen to many people with depressing regularity, but it was a new experience for me. I remember talking to the police, calling Bill to come collect me, and keeping on to the store on foot to buy something for dinner. I was still trying to operate in my super capable mode.

But when I faced a lot of complicated forms that had to be filled out, my resolve to keep calm failed. Arrangements had to be made for the car to be towed, mechanics and body shop people had to fit me in, two insurance companies had to haggle and estimate the damage. And I had to find a car to drive. For the most hardy souls these details can be frustrating and infuriating. Add to this the physical shock to my body which, while not even qualifying as whiplash, caused me to spend three days with every muscle aching. It was a run-of-the-mill accident. The car and I would mend. My capable period, however, became a thing of the past.

All of my responsibilities became too much. Dealing with insurance adjusters, trying to teach an active group of twelve-year-olds, being mother to three children, keeping the house

going were just too many balls in the air. They fell and I b
to fall apart too.

Cooking and housekeeping were the first to bite the du
stopped functioning and entered a whirlpool of helplessness
despair. I became incompetent, losing whatever I put down
often forgetting when I went upstairs why I had gone up t
My vision blurred even with glasses and reading was no lc
a pleasure. If I tried to call someone on the phone I could
a wrong number three out of four times. Everything insid
continually quivered. Food tasted strange, and my perceptic
the world totally changed. I felt alien, as though I'd never
in this place before and was completely ill-equipped to know
to navigate.

Everyday problems took on a nightmare quality. Bill w
tell me that we were a little short of cash this pay period a
immediately propelled myself into bagladydom, convinced t
would soon be roaming the city streets cold and penniless. 1
were no stages in my reactions. I went immediately to catastr
with no middle ground.

Somehow during that period I kept going to school wond
how long it would take for my co-workers and students to disc
my inability to cope. The students and I did learn to rec
very carefully the papers I marked as I made more than a
errors in correcting them. The kids were kind about it; I
perhaps it was a change to have a teacher who made errors
admitted them. It also meant that they had a fighting chan
improve the original grade on the paper. Incredible kids,
even reported mistakes that weren't in their favor. When tl
would reach the saturation point with me and I'd begin tc
teary, the children would sympathize, telling me tales of c
accidents and terrible treatment by insurance compa
Fortunately middle school children are old enough to empa
with someone they see hurting. I got lots of hugs and encourage
from them.

At home the family was puzzled and a bit frightened.
gone through a year of bad news, surgery, chemotherapy,
more surgery, but nothing like this had happened. Most frighte

was the fact that I closed up and had nothing to say. I was in such deep emotional pain that my strongest memory of that time was my wish to die quietly and end the agony for everybody. The closest I came to the idea of suicide was to try to use my self hypnosis and meditation to shut myself down permanently. This pain was unendurable.

I realize now that I am describing a clinical depression which sounds neat and classified. During my mental crash I called my doctors and they tried various medications to try to help me out of it. It seemed they had trouble believing that this formerly optimistic patient could swing so radically to the other end of the spectrum. So did I, but there I was. I could see no end to the pain, and finally realizing that I couldn't keep on like this, I sought the help of a professional therapist.

After the accident in October, Mom was very shaky. She wasn't hurt by the car that hit her, but she was angry about it. She had to spend hours on the phone trying to get the insurance company to have her car fixed. When she wasn't doing that she would go upstairs to her room and shut the door.

I don't remember who cooked dinner but I think Dad got stuck with it again. A lot of chores didn't get done but Mom didn't get mad like she usually does. She just seemed sad and quiet. She didn't go to P.T.A. She didn't want to do anything that was fun with me. She would just tell me, "It's too much; I can't." Everything was too much. Here she was, finally well and not even happy about it.

My favorite part of the year, the holidays, were coming up and that just seemed to make things worse. All I had to do was mention some little thing I wanted for Christmas and she would get mad. She'd tell me that she wasn't sure there would be a Christmas that year, she was too tired to go shopping and she didn't like Christmas anyway. A friend of Mom's invited our whole family to come to New York City for Christmas. He said that we could walk around Chinatown where they don't have Christmas and we could pretend it wasn't happening that year. The rest of the family said they were ready to go along with that

idea. That was the last straw for me. No Christmas. I (
and cried when I imagined no tree, no presents, no Chris
morning. It just isn't fair to take Christmas away from a
Finally Mom saw that I was right and said okay, we'd have
regular Christmas at home but we'd all have to help and it w
be much smaller than usual. I'd like to go to New York some
but on Christmas? You've got to be kidding.

On the one day in the fall when my teachers have mee
and my school is closed, Mom made me go with her to anc
hospital where she had an appointment with a therapist. She
she was having a hard time and was tired and discouraged.
said a therapist is something like a guidance counselor, somel
away from home that she could talk to. She had forgotten
I had the day off and told me I had to go with her because
needed to go and couldn't figure out a place for me to stay.
gave me a bag lunch and sat me in a little waiting room u
she went off for two hours. When she came back she looked
she'd been crying and wouldn't even stop for ice cream on
way home. Some day off.

PAT: Poor Ben. A day off and he had to spend it sitting in a wa
room. The therapist kept me a long time in the first sessio
walked in and the dam burst. I started from the beginning, u
most of her box of tissues as I sobbed and talked, realizing per
for the first time how much had happened to me in such a s
time. Finally after almost two hours, I got up to go and rea
I had no pocketbook with me. This was indicative of the w
was organizing my life at that stage. Panic set in as I imag
thieves at that very instant spending my money and using
credit cards. When I calmed down enough to make a phone
misdialing the number at least once, I found out that it was si
safely on my desk. I had apparently left my office with Ben
a car key. I was in rocky shape to face a resentful Ben who
been cooling his heels for two hours in a tiny reception area.
waited for praise and a reward for his patience and instead fc
himself herded to the car for a silent trip home. I didn't ca

In the weeks that followed, I had several more visits with my counselor who had been specially trained to deal with cancer patients. I began to understand how my grieving and anger had not really had time to be expressed and that now, when the active phase of treatment was complete, my mind needed time to understand and accept all that had happened. I'd been so busy holding my physical self together and trying to be Superwoman that I had completely run out of energy. What I needed most was time and I didn't see any way to find that. My counselor kept telling me to set priorities and I felt I had. I just was on overload in the priority department. If I left my job, I would be home with more time to think about my lousy luck. If I stopped making money I couldn't help Jeb go to college. If I didn't carpool Sean to driver's education, he would never drive and I would carpool forever. If I didn't take some interest in Ben's schoolwork, neither would he. If I left all the cooking and shopping to Bill, he would soon be in as bad shape as I was. Even writing this after a year, I can feel the panic and find myself wondering how we did survive, or frankly, whether we have!

Added to the logistics of survival and setting those damned priorities was the fact that the holidays were not far off. My illness had begun on Thanksgiving weekend and the mere thought of the holidays brought back in vivid detail all the painful memories of surgery and the possibility that I might die. If Christmas didn't come then somehow I wouldn't have to face those memories and the fact of my own mortality. To then think about gathering gifts and returning to our numerous Christmas traditions was out of the question. I cried some more.

On the advice of Anne Hahn, my therapist, I finally gathered my family together and told them how I was feeling. Ben was relieved that at least he didn't have to spend Christmas in Chinatown. The rest of the family were glad to be able to help in some way and agreed that a scaled-down Christmas was fine with them. Bill pointed out that I was the one who yearly escalated into crocheted snowflakes and elaborate cookies.

Still the holidays loomed as an impossible hurdle. Each day I'd think of what terrible event had occurred a year ago and relive

the misery with total recall. Anne and my doctor put me
mild anti-depressant which did make a big difference. I fi
accepted that I needed to experience this pain but I didn't
to wallow in it. If Xanax could get me through the holiday
swallow it.

Somehow Thanksgiving came and I didn't find another l
We went to my cousin's house for the annual gathering o
clan and devoured the traditional turkey followed by my cou
fabulous custom of baking at least eight different kinds of
My sister and her family were there also and Lee, knowing a
my panic over Christmas shopping, gave me a bag filled
beautiful quilted things she had made. This way she said I'd
presents to give out without the torture of shopping for t
Since deciding whether to cook hamburgers or hot dogs w
big decision at the time, it was a great relief not to have to
the holiday crowds. She, sensing my unhappiness, was gla
be able to do something concrete to help me survive this frighte
anniversary.

I began to take things very slowly, a small step at a time
this day I don't remember much about Christmas. I do remer
recycling the Christmas tree we used at school, which was a
three feet tall. The family gave me much good natured grief a
its size but it was easy to put up, trim and take down. I remer
thinking as I do each year that it was the prettiest one we'd
had. Somehow the stockings got filled and gifts appeared u
the tree. I only baked chocolate chip cookies instead of my u
elaborate assortment but that was okay. The kids really p
chocolate chip cookies. We had a quiet Christmas Eve sittin
the fire and reading Dylan Thomas's *A Child's Christmas in W*
We do that each year too, but it sounded better to me that Chris
than it ever did before. In a subdued way we tiptoed thr
the holiday season, all of us relieved that no further misfor
befell us.

BEN: *Before Mom's "crash" we had planned a trip to West Virg*
for Thanksgiving. We were supposed to stay with friends in
cabin in the mountains where it might even snow and we c

have an old-fashioned Thanksgiving and make gifts for Christmas. All of us were looking forward to getting away. Then Mom cancelled it. She said she couldn't go that far away, she was afraid of driving through the snow and she couldn't get organized.

We decided instead to have a work weekend at home. Sean made deer out of logs and sticks. I made hand-painted ornaments for the tree. Dad made big plans to build wooden cutting boards for people but never got around to making them. Mom and Jeb didn't do anything.

I was worried, by the way Mom was acting, that we wouldn't get any presents. She didn't go shopping and she didn't want to sit and plan Christmas like we did other years. She did keep going to her counselor and I hoped that she would help her.

Finally a sign of Christmas appeared on the pine chest in our dining room; two wrapped packages. They weren't for any of us but at least some presents were in the house and that meant that something must be happening. One weekend Mom got out a decorated basket we always put out at Christmas. It has Mr. and Mrs. Claus each holding up a side and it is usually full of candy or nuts. Well Mom put out the basket, but it stayed empty. I think one of her kids from school gave her candy for Christmas so it finally had something in it. Dad, who always says that Christmas is a nuisance, went out on his own and bought pine rope for our living room stairway. Mom didn't even ask him to. I got even more hope when Mom started to tell everybody how to hang the garland. Then she went to the attic and found more decorations and the favorite books we always read over the holidays.

Jeb came home from college, and it began to feel more and more like we would have a real Christmas. Jeb didn't have any money so he polished the brass rail around the fireplace. That made Mom happy. She was still telling everybody not to expect much, but she had gotten wrapping paper and there were more gifts on the pine chest. Jeb kept calling it the "no car, no money, three-gift Christmas."

Living in the country, we usually go out and cut down a tree, and it is always too big for our living room. Well, the one Mom brought home from her school was so small that she could carry

it in and set it up by herself. She plopped it down and to
that if anybody wanted a bigger one they could go get it.
one did, but we did tease her about her used tree. It took al
no time to trim, and we just used our most favorite ornam
I was glad to see any tree, but actually it really was just a p
little bush.

On Christmas Eve I helped Mom make braided Chris
bread. We went by to see friends and friends stopped by. It
snowed a little, which made it seem just right. Jeb and Sean
I were told to go to bed very early if we wanted Santa to c
That year I didn't put up any argument; I was too grateful
Santa was showing up at all.

Christmas morning looked like Christmas morning always
with presents all over the place. We each opened one at a
to make them last longer. I got to go first because I'm the you
and had the biggest pile. I got a boom box, models and
flannel sheets. Everybody got a toy because the family had r
a deal that everyone should always get a toy for Christmas.
year the older boys had just gotten clothes and tapes and
been really sad that none of their presents "did things" like
did. So now everybody gets wind-up toys or action figures,
Mom and Dad. Mom and I got our toy together. It u
dollhouse kit she had always wanted. She thought it woul
neat for me to build.

One funny thing about that Christmas was that the pack
from Santa had all the names mixed up. One brother got
shirts and the other got none. They just divided them up
but Jeb says he got shorted one package. The stockings we
little confused, and one kid would get three of something u
other people got none of it. No big deal, we just divided i
We realized that Santa didn't really have his act together, b
least he had shown up.

We had Christmas dinner at our friends' house. It was
like it always is. The table has a lace tablecloth and a little
with bows sits in the middle. At each place there is a tiny wo
angel or elf that holds a little candle. There is also a "crac
which is a paper firecracker that you don't light. You pull a s

and it pops. Inside is a prize, a riddle that is really dumb, and a paper hat that we wear at the end of Christmas dinner.

We got more presents and Roger, the father, said funny things that cracked everybody up. Roger always makes us laugh at Christmas dinner; that is part of our tradition. We had a big dinner, turkey, stuffing and finally the lights dimmed and in came the flaming Christmas pudding. You would think that is the end, but no. After the pudding we had mince pies, Stilton cheese, and port wine. The grown-ups let me have a small glass of wine that year.

We came home Christmas night and built a fire in the living room. I brought down my sleeping bag and pillow and we all sat and talked for a while. Then everybody went to bed, and I slept under the tree like I do every Christmas night. Christmas was back to normal.

After The Storm

The new year arrived, bringing with it a record snowfall, which left good friends snowed in with us for two days. What fun to watch the house and fields once more pile up with drifts as the crowd inside the house added logs to the fire, ate everything in sight and played Trivial Pursuit. We asked ourselves, "What will we do if the power goes out? What will we have for supper if this goes on for another day?" And most to the point for one dear friend, "What if my pipe tobacco runs out?" In Maryland where we live, it is fairly safe to ask these questions and feel sure that the snow won't last long enough to make it necessary to face the answers.

We figured out sleeping arrangements for family and guests and settled in "for a long winter's nap." When we awoke the world indeed was an impassable fairyland. The snow had lasted all night and was still falling gently. After a hearty breakfast and much toing and froing, we located snow gear and boots for most of the group. (In Maryland one never really expects snow and so never prepares for it.) We went outside, first to build a snowman with Ben, and then to pelt each other with snowballs. Finally the men and older boys got down to the serious business of gathering wood to keep our fire blazing. It was straight out of Norman Rockwell, with people looking rosy-cheeked and Sam, our dog, racing about, thoroughly enjoying the chilly novelty.

My friend Chrissi and I decided to take a walk down the farm road to look for deer tracks and to enjoy the experience of being the first humans on the snowy landscape. Sam joined us and we tripped and talked through the high drifts into the edge of the

wood. Suddenly Sam stopped and became rigid. We looke
at the ridge and saw the silhouette of a red fox against
background of the woods. All of us, even the fox, froze fc
instant, and I felt that moment of grace that comes to us v
something is perfect. Then Sam took off after the fox anc
fox did not run. Something was terribly wrong. The fox
caught in steel jaws hidden in the snow. Blood encircled hi
he tried in futility to escape the trap, the dog, and us. I s
horrified and heard myself screaming, "No No No."

Reality intervened. We first had to separate the furious
from the desperate fox. This I did with sticks while wild scre
came from depths of myself such as I had never heard. Ha
pulled the dog away, we started home for help, shaken and sadd
by what we'd seen.

There was nothing to be done. The farmer had the righ
set traps on his land; we were the trespassers. We went hom
sit by the fire and let the others deal with the animal out in
woods. It could have been our beloved dog who had wand
into the trap. It could have been Ben.

I could let this fox in his trap tear me apart, or I could ac
that we can't make the world safe, not for ourselves, the pe
we love, or a dying fox in the snow. We can do the best we
with what we're given or we can perpetually mourn for our lo
The choice at last seemed obvious.

BEN: *The first big snow of winter is the best and to have it on 1*
Year's Day was great. The guests were all grown-ups, but
kind who are fun to be around, so my brothers and everyl
got into the spirit of things. We had a snowball battle ana
in the snow and made angels. It was fun having everybody
over. The family got a VCR Clue game for Christmas ana
all played that. We got out all the cookies and ate them u
we played Trivial Pursuit. Mom was my partner. Dad coo
things and Mom cleaned up, but everybody was having fun.

Then Mom and Chrissi went out for a walk. They were g
pretty long and I went down the farm road to find them. N
came staggering up the road looking hysterical and telling me

to go down there and to go get Dad. Chrissi said there was a fox in a trap and not to go near because it might bite me. I got Dad and my brothers and we went down to see what we could do. There wasn't anything we could do; it was too late. Mom was so upset that I saw the fox. I had to explain to her that while I was sorry for the fox and I think traps like that should be against the law, I have grown up in the country and seen dead animals and blood. What bothered me most was that it made my mother so upset and almost ruined the first snow.

When we came back, Mom talked about it a little bit and we sat close for awhile. She was quiet and went to bed early that night, but that could have been because we'd had extra people and all the excitement. She talked to me after that about the fox, and we both seemed to understand that one person can't make everything work out. Sometimes sad things happen and that is the way it is.

Sometime in January I began to heal. No clouds parted, no orchestra played. I just quietly began marking papers correctly and miraculously reaching the phone number I dialed on the first try. I began to taste food again and enjoy the experience. I could drive home from work without getting panicky about fixing dinner. Still somewhat shellshocked, I didn't cheer. I just let the experience grow and hoped in a detached way that it would last. I was walking on eggs.

It was wonderful to pack up the Christmas ornaments and know that I had survived both holidays and was a year further from that wretched anniversary. We had even had some unexpected moments of peace and goodwill toward men, so often promised and so rarely delivered.

As school reopened, I remember walking down the hall thinking, "This is a good place; shopworn, but good." For the first time I saw how enthusiastic the children were, how much learning was going on. The imperfections and makeshift equipment faded into the background as I saw groups of children laughing and feeling good about themselves. Crumbling walls and grimy windows took their proper perspective. We were succeeding. Over the

months the walls were being covered with bright works of
All of us, students and teachers, had transformed this, the sch
into a warm, homelike place.

This is not to imply that we became a utopia of the mi
school world. We had crises and conflict on a minute to mi
basis. However, we had established a framework and a confid
in each other that helped us cope with the irate parent, the withdr
student, the missing bus, the lost carpool child. We even surv
the complexities of staging a full scale musical play, using
entire student body in the cast.

At home I still went to sleep around nine o'clock at n
Dinner was usually a joint effort with quite a few "do-it-your
nights thrown in. We kept a large supply of frozen pizza on h
Laundry and cleaning were done, but not very well. Dust bur
were more in evidence. Perfection was put on hold, and v
our shoes began sticking to the kitchen floor someone would
out the mop and swab the deck. On Saturday mornings w
tended to shrink away from the mess, but eventually we du
mopped and removed the week's massive collection of dog
junk mail and discarded clothing from the kitchen. We did
entertaining during that time. People stopped in and took u
we were. There was no other way.

As my therapist had said, over and over, one must set priori
Limits had to be accepted. I learned that dust will wait
somebody moves it. It just gets thicker. I learned to take s
time out. I was beginning to find that life does go on even
let go occasionally.

One thing we learned to do when the family reached
limits of frustration was to give each other a time out sign.
meant that no matter how ferocious the encounter we had to
and back off. While not bringing salvation, it did provide us
a way to avoid physical assault.

BEN: *Mom seemed happy with the way the new middle school*
going. I'd get to visit when my school closed and hers di
Ruxton Country School is very small; that year the whole mi
school had only thirty kids. The teachers joke with the kids

the kids get to use the computers almost every day. I used to go there when I was little, but Mom said it wasn't good for us always to be together, and in the middle school part she would have been my sixth grade teacher and my principal. That probably wouldn't have been a good idea. Still I do love to visit there.

My school was going okay. My grades were really good and I was asked to be part of the gifted and talented program next year in middle school. My behavior still wasn't the best. I have a problem sitting still and have always done my best work standing up and moving around. I've never been able to be quiet in school. That problem really has nothing to do with Mom. In fifth grade it was worse. I wasn't happy with my teacher and a lot of the work was boring. I think I am ready for a bigger school where they change classes and teachers. That way you get to move around and aren't stuck with the same teacher all day.

Mom seemed better than she had been. Winter was okay. We would snuggle and watch movies, and Mom would fall asleep. The difference now was that usually she'd stay asleep and we would tiptoe out of the room to give her a chance. Mom, Sean, and I could hope for snow days so we would get an extra day off. Snow days are the best days of the year. You don't plan snow days; you just wake up and hear the magic words "Baltimore County Schools will be closed today." Then, if you are sensible, you go back to sleep. I usually get up, wake Mom and tell her there's no school, and then go back to sleep if I can. Sometimes Mom makes me clean up my room on a snow day, but usually it is free time and hot chocolate.

This year Mom and I started building her dollhouse. I should say I started to help her, but there were all these little pieces and she wanted me to sand each one. I got splinters and she got grouchy and it wasn't much fun. I did know how to use the glue gun and helped with that part. Mom ended up building most of it herself, figuring out where all those little pieces went. I think it was good for her, as she had never built anything before. When she got to the part of putting in little windows, I was a big help. My hands are smaller than hers and I am much steadier. I've built models and had experience. Still, Mom did a great job

sanding, wallpapering and roofing. It took all of the winter
most of spring to finish it.

All in all we had a good winter. We went out some
people came to visit. Sometimes the family got fed up with
other, but I think that happens in every family. Besides the time
sign which we had agreed to use to stop a bad fight from happer
a friend told us about the word HALT. The letters stand
Hungry-Angry-Lonely-Tired. Before you lose your temper
say "Halt" to yourself and see if you are feeling one of t
things. Sometimes you can avoid trouble that way. Not alu
but it is a little like a time-out.

Everybody got a cold like we do most winters, which n
people cranky, but that was the worst that happened.

PAT: On one of those wonderful snow days, I opened the dollh
kit and was a goner. Inside were countless little wooden pi
and directions that promise, if followed correctly, all woulc
together and make a charming Victorian cottage. Ben looke
the small pieces, all of which needed careful sanding and pain
and the small print of the directions and decided it would be n
fun to go out and play in the snow. Bill politely refused t
roped into building it, reminding me that he was the one
had to cope with the idiosyncracies of our real Victorian cott
Sean agreed to act as consultant in emergencies and then
back to bed.

Ben returned to give it another shot from time to time,
usually ended up with a splinter in his finger or a cramp f
sanding. I also became very possessive and wanted it done
way.

Very gradually, in a painstaking way, I built a dollhouse. P
by piece, step by step I learned to slow down and discovered
constructing something is as much fun as admiring the finis
product. I learned to look at the world differently — in miniat
A drinking straw could become a lamp chimney, or a pretty bottle
an exquisite vase.

Sometimes I'd wake up in the middle of the night with
heart beating wildly and I'd lie in bed reliving the fear of

death. A nightmare might start the replay of my illness, which in the small hours of the morning would repeat itself endlessly. Some nights, I would get up and lose myself in fitting a tiny bay window, or stenciling miniature eaves. Whatever I did required total concentration and steady hands. Before long it was either morning or, more likely, I would be ready to return to bed and peaceful sleep.

As the dollhouse took on a recognizable shape, Ben rejoined the project and we had great times devising candles, shopping bags, tissue boxes and furniture. We have asked that Santa bring us a bigger one this Christmas, as Ben would like to create a game room with a pool table and a miniature dartboard he has already made. Ben thinks this new dollhouse is a strong possibility, as he has found a suspicious box in the garage.

Winter eventually did turn into spring and Ben and I once more checked the crocus crop and the progression of new growth in the garden. Another spring. I hadn't allowed myself to think that far ahead for a long while. Energy returned. Not the frenetic energy before I crashed, more like a lasting strength and a common sense approach. I wanted to take on more, but chose the activities I could handle. I joined a support group in Baltimore called NEED: Nutrition, Education, Exercise, and Discussion. There I met a group of women, all of whom had gone through the experience of breast cancer. We shared both the pain and our survival skills. The loneliness of what had happened to each of us was lessened.

Getting up my courage, I revisited Dr. McGibbon and set up a hospital date for the summer to complete my reconstruction and get a new nipple installed. I rented a house at the beach where we could all go and finally have our overdue vacation. I signed up for a summer course at a college away from home where I would learn about managing a middle school. Ben and I decided to write a book. I realized that I am prone to hyperactivity unrelated to my illness and that I have to learn to live with it. I wanted to do all the things I set up for this summer. I was being self-indulgent. I was finally letting go.

On With The Show

: A*nother summer is about to end and I am getting ready to start back to school next week. This school doesn't want you to get your school supplies until you meet with each of your teachers. Another tradition gone, but Mom says we can go shopping anyway for some shoes and a binder and paper. I am starting the sixth grade in the new middle school in my neighborhood. I'll be in the same grade that Mom teaches. When I went with Mom before to visit her class, I always felt like a little kid. Not anymore.*

It has been a good summer. We actually got a vacation and went to the beach. My friend Joey went with us. We let Mom hold our money. We didn't blow it all at once like we used to. We decided how much to take each day when we went to the boardwalk and that was all we'd spend.

There are changes in me and most of them are for the better. I used to spend every penny I had whenever I got a chance and then bug Mom for more. I used to get very mad and have temper tantrums. Then I would run away or hide, like I did when Mom was in the hospital. One time I ran away and got lost. I wouldn't do that anymore. Now when I am very angry with my mother and father I go to my room and cool down, or I go out for a walk, but I do let them know I am going.

When Mom was sick I did steal some things from her. I have always liked to sneak into my brothers' rooms and borrow stuff. But this was different. I took all kinds of things, some I didn't need, like jewelry, pens, candy and money. I think I did it partly to get back at Mom for getting sick. The money was a little different; I just wanted lots of it. I thought it would make everybody feel better. I used some of the money I took to buy Easter pre for my mom and dad. Still, whatever the reason, it was w for me to take it. I gave most of the stuff I took back and Mom what I had done. I don't want to be a thief, and no m what excuse you think you have, you do not take things other people or go through their drawers. As for my brothe am beginning to understand how they feel and I have sto going into their rooms unless I am asked. I'm not sure I'll r sneak around again because they have some really neat stuff even now I sometimes get tempted.

I could blame what I did on Mom getting sick, but I think that is fair. Kids do some rotten things sometimes they are growing up, and I think I am a pretty normal kid. I can try to do is stop the bad behavior and remember sometimes I might slip up. Nobody's perfect.

Mom has been great this summer. She has acted more she used to, and I feel like I can depend on her again like th days. She did go back to the hospital, but it was only for night. A week later she was back on her feet doing wha does. All of us are glad she doesn't have to have more sur The cancer could come back; that is one of the reasons cano such a horrible disease. Mostly I don't think about that. W the point? Mom is well now, but she could get sick again. No knows for sure what will happen. I just learned sooner than kids that my parents don't have all the power. They can't al be sure what is going to happen to them. They want to their children safe, but they can't even do that all the time makes me sad and it makes me angry that this is true, b doesn't change things. The idea that my mother could die m me lonely and frightened. I still need her too much.

If Mom did have a recurrence, she would do chemothe again or maybe some other treatment. I'm glad that there treatments for her. I hope I'd be more of a help about it, I'm not really certain. I am older now and would try to unders but a person never knows for sure how they would act until have to. I mean I didn't think when I was a goalie that I w *dive for the ball like I sometimes did. You can disappoint yourself sometimes, but you can surprise yourself too.*

Most kids don't think too much about death. Most of the time when they do it is pretend, like G.I. Joe or playing war where everyone gets up afterward and keeps on playing. I have learned more about death. I learned that all of us will die someday and that if you are very old or your body has suffered a terrible disease or accident that death isn't the worst thing that can happen. I don't want my family or pets to die. None of our animals have ever died. Some of our friends have, though.

The same weekend that Mom found the lump, I went to a funeral. Lyn, a good friend of our family, was the first dead person I had ever seen. I didn't have to look, but I wanted to. I couldn't believe it. I waited for her to get up and give me a hug like she always did. I hoped she would tell me it was all a joke, but she didn't. I don't want to die but I am not too scared about it. I just hope I am a very old man when it happens. Really though, I don't think about it much. There is too much to do that is a lot more fun.

Finally we got away to the beach and it was perfect. We shared a house with our best friends and had time to walk, sit on the beach, talk, and, at least three times a day, indulge ourselves in what Bill called a "feeding frenzy." We got to read, swim, ocean watch, fly kites, or just sit if that was what we felt like doing. How seldom we get the chance to do what we want when we want to. And for a whole week. It flew by and we returned to a broken dishwasher, a crippled car, and the chaotic version of housekeeping that our older sons had adopted.

The rest of the summer was spent learning to use a computer and walking. The first had intimidated me, since the kids brought home their first Atari and I had trouble with Pac-Man. My husband is a computer analyst and his sophisticated explanations scared me even more. Now I wanted to organize all the material Ben and I had gathered for this book, and the computer seemed the most practical way. Finally, with help from Jeb, Sean, Bill, and

Ben, I learned enough to type, print, and save what I intend
type, print and save. Most of the time.

The entire family was so pleased when a day arrived wi
my needing someone to come sort me out of some incre
scramble I'd created. I've learned to respect what these mac
can do, knowing how little I know about them. It has also
good to learn something new and rediscover that my minc
still function, something I wasn't sure of for awhile.

I recovered enough stamina and had enough time this sur
to attempt to do something about the state of my body. I
in a sorely neglected condition, as chemotherapy and surger
left me too tired and unmotivated for physical exercise. A
best of times my approach to fitness is sporadic, and durin
illness, my exercise program consisted of walking arounc
short circular driveway and, on good days, taking a ten-m
stroll down the farm road. Now I began to walk in earnest.
loves an outing, and all I had to do was whisper the magic
"walkies" and he would spring into action, ready for anyt
The rest of the family did not share his enthusiasm, so Sar
I would set off alone at 6:00 A.M. when it was cool and
for about an hour. At first we didn't go far in the time allc
but we have now worked up to a speed of about four mil
hour, interrupted by Sam's frequent stops to answer the ca
nature. I can feel my body firming up a bit and my energy
increasing. I haven't figured out how to manage these walks
school reopens and the weather turns cold and dark. They
become important, a matter of setting priorities again. M
I'll take up mall walking.

In August I went back to the hospital for my pre-op te
before going in to have my nipple reconstructed. I was prou
the way I drove there, parked and went in without too r
butterflies doing a number on me. I breezed through the b
work, EKG, and insurance interview, reminding myself: it's
a one-night stand and I'll be coming home with a nipple.
bad can that be? I went in for the routine physical exam
was feeling pleased at my low blood pressure and slow pulse
when the doctor told me she could feel a small lump on my s

and thought she had better inform my surgeon. I immediately re-entered that twilight zone where one hopes for a quick simple explanation, but fears having to gear up to face a new crisis. I no longer experience denial when a suspicious lump is found. I also, having had several lumps in the last year, do not plan my funeral and settle my affairs. I put myself on hold and wait for the second and maybe even third opinion while going through whatever tests are required. Each time brings back some of the terror and despair of my original encounter with cancer. This is the tightrope walked by every former cancer patient. We know the statistics, we know the tenacity of the disease. Cancer is a part of our past and, checking the odds, could be a part of our future. We become cliff dwellers, enjoying our elevated view while being aware of the uncertainty of our tenure. Each lump, each setback, is a threat, but we can't afford to overreact. Our balance is too precarious.

As soon as I got home from the hospital I called my surgeon, who reassured me that my lump was probably nothing, but that he would certainly check it out when I came in for the operation. Two days I had to wait and wonder about this latest development. I called my oncologist. As he had seen me not long before, he too reassured me that the lump was probably a cyst and not malignant. He promised to check it out when I got to the hospital. I decided that both doctors were in a state of denial and couldn't yet cope with my latest recurrence.

By the time I was admitted, my lump was larger and had begun to itch. Dr. McGibbon quickly diagnosed it as a mosquito bite. Oh my God, two days of hanging in an iron cage over a mosquito bite! Dr. Padgett's second opinion confirmed this, and he added that one can feel pretty safe about bumps and lumps that itch. Malignant tumors do not. Off I went to have my nipple restored, feeling greatly relieved, but not so convinced that I didn't ask for the area to be rechecked after the "malignant mosquito bite" was gone. Who knows, maybe there was a lump under the bite. There wasn't.

The surgery required only one night in the hospital and a week in an elastic-harness-corset-type bra to keep things from

moving. When finally unveiled, the nipple looked a bit large
my doctor promised me that it would eventually shrink and m
its counterpart. When I look in the mirror without my gla
they match perfectly. In October I go in to get it tattooe
color so it will be identical. Then reconstruction will be comp
That is a good feeling.

Tonight I am going to my support group of friends who
all had mastectomies. We all touch base from time to time,
some of them will want to see this latest addition to my
breast. Reconstruction is not for everybody, and I think
better to wait until the trauma of the mastectomy has rec
and you are sure you want to do it. Some people want to a
elective surgery altogether, and I can certainly understand
point of view. I just needed to put things back as I thought
should be. For me it was something I could do to help put i
behind me. Now I can present a united front to the world.

My recuperation complete, I am about to face the begin
of a new school year. Jeb has left the nest again for his ju
year at college. Sean, Ben and I are running around clearing
our rooms. Bill says we have PSS (Pre School Syndrome).
particularly edgy and want to see the house clean, the toma
canned, the bills paid, and the children with new shoes and hair
And I want all this to happen at once. The summer is over, f
routines must be restored. I am deep cleaning, a sure sign
energy is about to be shifted to school and I won't tackle
cobwebs here for a long time.

I am still walking, eating, and trying to lose weight. I
reading, writing, and healing. Occasionally I am crying and ha
nightmares. I wonder about the second anniversary and fa
the holidays. I am glad to be around and well so I can da
wonder about those things.

Ben and I have a date to go on a tour of his new mi
school and get him fitted for his gym suit. After that we'll
for the mall for his annual back to school outfits and sc
supplies. Maybe we'll go out to lunch. Why not splurge?

After Mom's last trip to the hospital, she came home and helped me get ready for camp. Yes, camp. We found another one not far from home, which is great. The kids my age live in an Indian village and the cabins aren't cabins; they are different Indian dwellings like tepees, long houses, and a Navajo hogan. I was assigned to the hogan, which is an eight-sided building with a hole in the roof so you can build a fire inside it and lie on your bunk and watch it.

When I first arrived at Camp Puh'Tok, I met a shy boy who was moving into the hogan. It was his first time away from home, and even though I was new to this camp, I tried to help him get used to being away. The hogan filled with kids and we all got along with one another. The counselors came from all over the place; England, Spain, Germany, Scotland, and Baltimore. The camp had great activities and I really didn't have time to get homesick. Most of the things we did had to do with Indian traditions. Some of the things were challenges that Indian boys had to do to become part of this tribe. There are steps to manhood, and I took the first one by staying in a sweat lodge. That is a log cabin with a canvas floor. Under the floor are rocks which are very hot. The counselors pour hot water on the rocks and the lodge feels like it must be 1000 degrees inside. Six of us stayed inside until the time was up. I felt very strong to be able to do that.

I learned lots of other things at camp, like Indian lore, archery, lacrosse, and black powder musketry. I was glad to see Mom and Dad at the closing campfire, but I can't wait to go back next year.

I have grown up a lot in the last two years, maybe a little faster because Mom did get sick. I still have some problems and I sometimes feel afraid without really knowing why. Starting in a new school makes me scared, and I have been sick to my stomach off and on for a couple weeks. It makes me feel so alone when my stomach is upset. I don't know how Mom stood it all those months.

Sometimes I sleep on the floor of my parents' room. I s
is because they have air conditioning, but it is partly that I
better being close to them. Maybe by the time the furnace
on I'll be ready to sleep alone. My room is pretty cold, the

Still I don't think I am as insecure as I was. Insecu
someone who sleeps with the lights on and refuses to try
things. Even though there are times when I feel like I can
something I am usually brave and do it anyway. If you are
insecure you sometimes punish other people because you c
think much of yourself. I am pretty proud of myself for stic
with Mom and helping out. I am stronger and taller now
am very helpful around our place. I can drive the tractor
mow the grass; I can reach the tall cabinets and put things a
And I clean things, sometimes without even being asked. I k
I am needed to keep things going. I was the baby of the fa
for a long time, and it was fun. Now, though, I am ready t
more grown up. It doesn't mean I can't hug people or play
be silly; it just means that I understand more about how c
people feel and how some kids have times even rougher th
did. I still have my mother and father, they still love each c
and me, and we are all together.

You can't ask for more than that.

CHAPTER 11

Bill's Chapter

When you walk in the mountains with all you need on your back, at first it is impossible to see anything, to enjoy anything, because of your aching legs and shoulders. Sooner or later the miraculous body-mind machine adapts to the challenge, the solid lead backpack somehow becomes bearable, and then you can start to have some fun. The exhilaration of being your own boss, being free and *coping* is destroyed in an instant by a serious injury, a badly sprained ankle. Or a close brush with death. Now you, or a fellow traveler, may not make it to the end, much less carry all that weight. The loads will have to be redistributed among the others, and most likely something will have to be left behind.

When Pat got sick, we all picked up as much of the burden as we could. All of us found we could bear heavier stress longer than we had imagined, but I think Ben had almost as bad a time as Pat because it was his first big-time crisis. He didn't *know* how to deal with panic, how to revel in a current good moment while shutting out all the bad stuff, how to wring seeds of hope from a bleak situation, or many other coping techniques which life had given the rest of us opportunity to learn. He learned fast, and came through this very difficult time with honor and fortitude. The physicians gave Pat a fighting chance and more, but sometimes, when everything seemed hopeless and she felt about ready to give up, I believe Ben was the main reason that she kept trying.

Some of our friends read the early drafts and felt that Jeb, Sean and I should have gotten more space. It is true that I could not have managed without their help, Pat and I both recognize

their contribution and its value. Perhaps all those alarms
excursions of ours during this period *would* make a good s
but *this* book is about learning to cope with crisis, and the
no doubt that Ben and Pat learned the most, since their
were the hardest hit.

We are ready to resume our journey. Rather than go
the way they came, however, I like to think that Ben and
have decided to keep on wherever the path may lead, lea
behind this cairn of words and feelings. Others who must t
this way will see it and know that somebody made it this
stopped for a while, and then went on to see what was ar
the next bend of the trail.

BILL BRACK

Three Years Later

Way back when I was rocking my first baby, sometime around 3:00 A.M., I decided I had no need of lofty ambitions; it would be enough if I could raise my children in as sane a way as I could in a world full of uncertainties and problems. At the time it seemed a very basic and humble ambition. It is not so simple. I've had to learn my limitations and repeatedly accept that I can't make the world safe for my family. They in turn don't expect me to and get impatient when I revert to trying. It is important that we have time together to go to the beach, get the grass cut, and the tomatoes canned, that we can sit together on our old screened porch to talk of our mutual trials and recall past thunderstorms.

Ben has just spent the morning packing his footlocker for his third summer at Camp Puh'Tok. He is talking about becoming a counselor-in-training (depending upon the benefit package) and can't wait to be away from lawn mowing and parental supervision. Gone are the days when I would pack him up from a sheaf of carefully compiled lists, making sure he had bug repellent and a new stuffed animal to keep him from being eaten and lonely, respectively. This year I am not sure what he has in that trunk, though I have glimpsed sour-cream-and-onion potato chips and a bag of powdered sugar doughnuts. I doubt he has remembered to pack socks or toothbrush but it is some measure of how much he has grown up that he took the initiative and got himself ready for camp.

Ben has had a busy time going from ten to thirteen years
He is a delightfully infuriating blend of arrogance, vulnerab
bravado, sweetness and fun. He curses more than he whi
these days, but he has maintained a sense of humor despite
(and new) pressures. Noisy, active, lazy, and enthusiasti
challenge to parents and teachers, Ben has experienced (and sh
with his family) most of the traumas such a transition requ
He has abandoned teddy bears for a Walkman radio and
music. He no longer sleeps on the floor of our room, has ta
to doing things for himself, and decides more often exactly
he wants his life to be.

BEN: *I've just finished reading the galleys for our book and it
sometimes as if I was reading about someone I'd never met.
changed an awful lot from the little boy in fourth and fifth gi
to a pretty grown up eighth grader. Not only have I gotten t
and less dumpy, but my interests have changed too. Things
algebra and girls. I look back at the things I did when I was
and feel a little ashamed and embarrassed about some of it.
when I think back to that cold and forbidding hospital roor
still understand why I freaked out and hid under the chair
ran up and down the hall. I bet some adults feel like doing
same thing in a hospital; they are just too afraid to do it.
not so grown-up that I can't remember what it feels like to
kid.*

PAT: Over the past three years our family settled, at first unea
into a new normal routine as my strength returned. We addre
some of the less pressing problems of life: blossom end-rot on
tomatoes, poison ivy in the flower garden, broken appliances
frayed clutch cables, and the ever-present leaky plumbing
falling paster.

There were many times when my episode with cancer see
so far away in the past that it might have happened to some
else. Marking the uneventful anniversaries of discovery
treatment gave me more confidence every year. I plunged
the present with all the energy I had, actually more plunging

not enough energy. By May of 1988, I had again overextended myself and was beginning to wear out.

Many cancer survivors seem to feel that we must affirm over and over our survival and recovery, that we must crowd as much as we can into each day, that if one is to accomplish anything worthwhile it should be started immediately and finished as soon as possible. Nothing important can be put on the back burner.

Some aspects of this were energizing and exciting. I seemed to have a heightened perception of time, of the season, and of possibilities for myself, my family, and the new middle school. I loved having the chance to develop our school, to work with people who want to humanize education. Life was so busy that I neglected the activities that helped me recover from chemotherapy and surgery. Instead of meditation and daily walks, I pushed myself, despite the return of gradually increasing insomnia, fatigue, and arrhythmia.

I was becoming apprehensive, afraid of another crash, and needed help: I had won the big fight but needed something more. I needed to calm down. A middle school parent who is a practicing psychiatrist noticed my semi-frantic efforts to run the middle school, teach her son, keep my family going and still maintain an optimistic attitude about my former medical problems. She took me aside and kindly suggested acupuncture, which she had found helpful in a post-surgery situation.

I decided to try it. I had doubts at first: I didn't understand how acupuncture treatment worked, and the idea of being stuck with little needles is not very attractive after extensive treatment with the larger variety.

In late May I went to Alice Camara at the Baltimore Center for Traditional Acupuncture. Alice is a gentle, no-nonsense RN and Registered Acupuncturist. My first session was preceded by a thorough physical by an M.D. and did not, to my relief, include any needles. Then for an additional two hours Alice took a complete history, listening not only to the medical facts and details, but taking the time to find out how I felt about all of the adjustments my body and soul had had to deal with in such a short time.

Her attention, sympathy, and concern were therapeutic
themselves. I began weekly treatment.

The improvement was not noticeable at first. It was so gen
so all-encompassing, that only gradually did I become aware
I was feeling better. Acupuncture ultimately restored a m
needed peace to my life. I still return for "booster" shots w
overwhelmed by busy days and unavoidable stress.

By Christmas that year I was feeling relaxed and read
enjoy the return home from college of our two older sons.
modified the holiday partying and skipped the yards and y
of pine rope which annually dropped needles everywhere.
did recreate our tradition of original and famous gingerb:
people, including the inevitable bikini-clad, big breasted pin
Ben mixed the dough and it was the best tasting we've ever l
Once again we tortured Bill with the absolute worst Christ
music, courtesy of our local gas station which offered a cass
for $2.98 even if you didn't buy gas.

I purposely scheduled my annual mammogram after
holidays, reasoning that never again would I combine Christ
and cancer if I could possibly avoid it. February seemed the
time to go.

I did not pass my mammogram. My radiologist was c
again sad, kind, and hesitant as he told me that the results v
'worrisome'. He recommended a biopsy as soon as possible, ha
detected small abnormalities which he said may or may not l
been malignant. The biopsy was immediately set up for the
of the week.

I went home feeling hopeful that a) it wasn't malignant,
b) even if it was it would be so small that the surgeon co
remove it all during the biopsy and that would be the end of
glitch in my back-to-normal life. Only at 2:00 or 3:00 A.M.
my thoughts turn desperate. Any abnormality is scary and
track record was not the best. Only in the middle of the n
could I allow myself the thought of another possible mastect
and all that it could involve.

During the biopsy I remained awake, cheerful, and optimi
My surgeon was being so thorough as he carefully removed

worrisome areas, excising the old scar tissue from the earlier reconstruction. He stitched so delicately—surely this was the end of the matter?

The news from the pathology lab, however, was both good and bad. More extensive microscopic tests showed I had a new primary malignancy in the earliest stages; a second modified radical mastectomy was recommended.

The good news was that the cancer was not a recurrence. The original more invasive cancer had not travelled to the right breast and the chemotherapy looked as if it had done its job and prevented metastasis. More encouragement followed when the doctors explained that it was unlikely I would need chemotherapy as the malignant cells were so small and well-contained. The new high resolution/low radiation machines can pick up problems that might have grown for years without being detected by breast self-examination or by less sophisticated x-ray/mammogram equipment.

The surgery was scheduled as soon as possible, for the next week. Having a previously assembled SWAT team of doctors who knew me and whom I trusted made these decisions less frightening. I met with my reconstructive surgeon who felt that because of the unlikelihood of chemotherapy he could perform the breast reconstruction immediately following the mastectomy. This now seemed like wonderful news; I would only have to ride into the O.R. one time, only endure one bout of anesthesia. I had begun to accept these new terms for survival.

Ben was angry. His original response was straightforward and ticked off. "Not again," I think, were his initial words as he grabbed the dog, retreated to his room and slammed the door. He was not interested in details or explanations; he had done this once and wanted no part of a repeat performance. I got angry too and marched into his room to inform him that like it or not, I had a few more hurdles to jump, not just as his mother, but as me. I told him that I'd do it and do it well with or without him, but it would make things easier if we worked at it together rather than battling each other. I wished him a night of severe insomnia for being such a pain and left. He went to sleep.

Thirteen is very different from nine, especially f[
thirteen-year-old who has had three years to face the fact tha
mother is mortal. I felt more in control and somewhat ca
this time and thus I was able to reassure the family that th
didn't look as grim; I fully intended to make this surger
uneventful as possible so we could all return to business as u

After Ben's initial anger and denial he went along with
inevitable and decided to get me through. He sent me a
saying so and the night before surgery Ben, Bill and I had
evening out eating Chinese food. Bill and Ben each presented
with a miniature light fixture for the doll house along with a
reassuring me that I light up their lives. We ate too much, laug
and enjoyed our time together. We have learned
compartmentalize. It is pointless to give up the good times.

The surgery went smoothly, helped by massive support
friends. After five days in the hospital I went home,
reconstructed breast complete except for the nipple. Bill and
decided to keep the home front as quiet and normal as poss
and with friends supplying food and encouragement the disrup
at home were minimal. Ben remembered the routine from
other hospitalizations and arranged flowers, provided ice w
and a way for me reach it, unpacked my bags and kept me comp
for a day or two after which, assured that I would make i
returned to his normal round of activities, coming in for
visits but otherwise busy.

BEN: *When Mom got cancer again, I was mad at first. I felt
I'd already been through hell coping with it the first time
now I was going to have to do it all over again. I didn't g
thought to how Mom was feeling and how it must have hurt
I just didn't want anything to do with it. Eventually when
used to the idea, I also realized that there were things I coul
to help out and that if I did, the whole thing might go bette
all of us. Being older I was able to help by taking phone
and letting her sleep, bringing her coffee or water and mostly
of hugs and kisses to let her know that we cared and to pu
in a fighting mood.*

We got through the second operation pretty well with Mom busy seeing her friends and working on her dollhouse stuff. I was busy being on another championship indoor soccer team. Mom knew she didn't need chemotherapy this time and she wouldn't have to go back to the hospital for reconstruction and I think that helped too. It just wasn't as scary for any of us as the first time. Maybe you can just get used to anything but I think my mom had grown very strong and this made the rest of us feel stronger too. Sometimes, even early on I forgot that she had been sick at all.

My recovery was uneventful, I believe in part because we realized this was not a repeat of the first time and we had our priorities in order. I took the time to rest and didn't feel the need to prove my strength and survival to family and friends. I continued the acupuncture treatments which helped me maintain my balance and even enjoy the quiet healing time. I admitted the stiffness from the back muscles involved in the reconstruction and went to physical therapy for heat treatments and massage. Cancer isn't very easy to deal with but all of us had developed some survival skills. We learned patience as we waited for test results and healing. No one, including me, expected me to be a superwoman. Bill and I kept our sense of humor and learned that humor is one of Ben's primary ways of getting through life.

He won a contest at his school for the funniest head by gluing a model helicopter, tanks and army men in his hair.

He made me laugh by putting hangers inside his clothes, over his ears, and pretending to be a closet.

We got numerous reports from teachers about Ben's perpetual clowning and unwillingness to take school seriously. Although we would like Ben to settle down I was secretly glad that his reaction to the events at home was to try to make people laugh. He could have turned sullen, withdrawn, gotten into fights—who knows? At least his misbehavior was an attempt to make someone happy. The coach of Ben's first place undefeated soccer team told us that Ben's unfailing cheerfulness, spirit and sense of fun was a major contribution to the team. Good news. Our son is a survivor.

BEN: *By the time seventh grade was ending I was ready for my fis*
pole and summer days exploring the woods with my dog .
Most exciting of all was the fact that our whole family, all
of us, was taking a trip to England. I had never been out o
country before. The second to last school day I bounded of
school bus for the last time that year. I ran faster than I
thought I could go to our front porch, jumped onto the p
and greeted all three cats with a loud "HELLO." Then stra
outside to help Mom, Dad, and Sean pack the car for the ric
the airport. I got my last minute important stuff like tapes
my Walkman and an extra pair of underwear, and we were

We spent a long night on the plane and woke up with Heath
Airport below us. I couldn't believe it. So many wonderful t
we had. I'll never forget walking into Hamley's Toy Stoi
London. Suddenly I was four years old again and I never,
wanted to leave that place.

PAT: I prepared for our trip to London with extra acupunc
treatments and physical therapy and off we went to a tiny
floor walk-up flat for twelve days. In short order we rea
that this was not the dream vacation we had envisioned a
struggled very much together through a heat wave, a tube/rai
strike, and no two people ever being hungry, sleepy or in
mood for Westminster Abbey at the same time. We argued
enjoyed, we tested our legs and our stamina. We saw the Tc
of London, the noisy streets of SoHo, and the fireworks or
Thames for the Queen's birthday celebration. We travelled thr
the Cotswolds and Wales by car as Sean navigated and Bill mast
the aggressive art of the round-about and the M-4 motorwa

Ben and I walked arm in arm through the London Dun
and Warwick Castle. He sat patiently through a very long,
production of Shakespeare's *Cymbeline* in Stratford. We to
short nap on the grassy floor of the ruins of Tintern Abbey.
five of us had time together without all the responsibilitic
being home. We were all learning a new place and I w
participant, not the problem. Yes it was tiring, maybe I sh

have waited until I was stronger, but I was feeling good and wanted to share an adventure with my family. Most mothers want their children to be strong and self-sufficient. I have perhaps a greater sense of urgency in wanting them to try out their wings. It was great to see how capable all of them are, being able to navigate the streets and underground system in London, to unearth the best pub lunch, or find the complicated route through the mountains of Wales. They were confident and it was a relief to trust them with some of the responsibility.

For the whole trip I never thought about how Mom had been sick and I don't think she did either. There were just too many things to do. Then, in Wales, we got some news that brought us down to earth with a thud. We got a call from home saying our dog Sam was dying and probably would not make it through the night. That call brought back everything and Mom and I went out to the garden and cried. Then I knew that if Mom died I wouldn't know what to do. If I could bring Sam or Mom back with my love I would but I know we can't always do that. I know that we should give the people and animals we have all the care and loving we can while they are here so that if we do lose them we will know we have done our best. By the way, Sam was very sick and the vet said many times that he probably wouldn't make it, but he is here running around and getting into the garbage. Doctors aren't always right.

Now we are back at home and I am almost finished with middle school. Our family still has its ups and downs mostly over teenager things like my dirty room, too much television, homework and what I should wear. Like why I couldn't go downtown in a wrinkled tee shirt and torn jeans. From my point of view I'm just expressing myself. Mom truly is stronger than she's ever been which means I don't get away with as much any more. I still manage to watch too much TV, blast my music and never hear my parents when they are calling me to do chores.

Our family is changing, Jeb lives away from home now and Sean is gone a lot at college. I am an only child and while I miss my brothers there are some advantages to being the only kid. I get a larger piece of coffee cake in the morning, and more *in the shower. Only two people tell me what to do instea* *four. I've gotten stronger, too.*

PAT: Ben has grown up and doesn't need to be tucked in most nig Sometimes he'll allow me to curl up on the bed to discuss latest plane and collections (key rings, coins and mugs at moment). Most of Ben's homework is done on his own. H often out with friends and spends much of his time at h listening to his stereo, taking showers, and being deaf to requ to take out the trash. His idea of heaven would be a phone a TV in his room and a slot in his door through which n could be deposited. Ben is on track. For almost four year has grown up with a mother who had serious medical probl Like it or not, this is part of his definition of what his moth Ben has cemented his relationship with his dad far more than brothers had at his age and will often turn to Bill first whe has a crisis. Bill in turn has taken over more of the nurtur It is both a relief and a comfort to me that the responsibili shared.

BEN: *I hate to see our traditions change. I was worried about Christ* *this past year because Jeb couldn't stay with us very long. I n* *wanted Christmas to change. As it turned out, this was the* *Christmas I ever had. Instead of being a little kid, I really sh* *the jobs like untangling tree lights and mixing MY recipe* *gingerbread men. Feeling the love in our house at Christmas* *would make any old miser smile. My brothers both came h* *and I had a TV we were giving Jeb under the presents (he fig* *it out). I sneaked a CD player that all three of us boys go* *my father into my room and hid it. It wasn't just the sneak* *that made me feel good but the fact that I am a grown-up men* *of this family now at last. I had a chance to plan surprises* *make other people happy. I dreamed of years to come wh* *have children, and their Grandmother Brack helps me make* *Christmases as exciting as all mine were. Families are what all about and ours is more than okay. I am thankful for my family, and especially my mom.*

I was proud but not surprised this past Christmas to see Ben gleefully planning all of the festivities, taking over the standard parental jobs of baking and buying presents. If Ben had learned anything from our experiences, it was the value of family relationships, and every gift he gave and every gesture he made were full of affection. And, although he was sad to see his brothers go, Ben was able to face the realities of his family's comings and goings as well as the warmth of the times together. Ben and I are back in business. Life is once more full of possibilities.

PAT BRACK

BIBLIOGRAPHY

Benson, Herbert, with Miriam Z. Klipper. *The Relaxation Response.* New York: William Morrow & Co., 1975; New York: Avon Books, 1976.

Bruning, Nancy. *Coping with Chemotherapy.* New York: Ballantine Books, 1985.

Connelly, Diane M. *All Sickness Is Home Sickness.* Columbia, Maryland: Center for Traditional Acupuncture, 1986.

Hazelton, Lesley. *The Right To Feel Bad.* New York: Ballantine Books, 1984.

Herzfeld, Gerald and Powell, Robin. *Coping For Kids.* West Nyack, New York: The Center For Applied Research in Education, Inc., 1986.

LeShan, Lawrence. *How To Meditate.* Boston: Little, Brown, 1974; New York: Bantam Books, 1975.

Simonton, O. Carl, Stephanie Matthews-Simonton and James Creighton. *Getting Well Again.* Los Angeles: J.P. Tarcher, 1978; New York: Bantam Books, 1984.

Siegel, Bernie S. *Peace, Love and Healing.* New York: Harper & Row, 1989.

————. *Love, Medicine and Miracles.* New York: Harper & Row, 1986.

Sterns, Ann Kaiser. *Coming Back.* New York: Random House, 1988.

Viorst, Judith. *Necessary Losses.* New York: Simon and Schuster, 1986.

Pat Brack, a native of Maryland, has spent most of her professional life teaching at Ruxton Country School in Baltimore. The middle school division, which Pat established in 1986, currently operates with fifty-two students and attempts to convince children they need not be miserable to be educated. Pat serves as head of the middle school, teaches creative writing, supervises admissions, does counseling, organizes placement of graduates, assists with school plays and washes the faculty coffee pot.

At home Pat enjoys walks through the country with the dog and anyone else who will join her. She collects and creates miniatures and is filling her house with dollhouses and habitats. Pat avoids housework and is always thinking about getting her closets straightened. She would much prefer to travel, preferably to Europe or the beach, any beach.

She currently lives in White Hall, Northern Baltimore County with husband Bill, sons Jeb, Sean and Ben, three elderly cats and a dog named Sam.

Ben Brack is now fourteen and looking forward to graduation from eighth grade at Hereford Middle School. Ben has survived being the youngest of three brothers and finds the sports of soccer and lacrosse relaxing alternatives.

The young author has many talents and interests including painting, model construction, loud music, building things and earning money. He enjoys his annual escape to camp in the summer. Ben is working to become fluent in French so he can call the shots if the family ever returns to Europe. His long term plan is to attend St. Mary's College in Maryland.

Ben still gives his mother a hard time though he loves her very much.

Reach to Recovery

Just about the time the anesthesia was wearing off after my mastectomy, I began to be aware of all the practical problems involved in getting on with my life. My first attempt to move my arm and reach for something was a shock as my shoulder was stiff and sore and no movement could be taken for granted. There were new sensations I hadn't really anticipated, like the feeling of lead weights hanging from the chest and arm giving an unpleasant feeling of heaviness. I was a bit muddled from the surgery and, once the dressings were changed and the new terrain uncovered, there was the problem of ever looking or feeling normal again. The medical personnel looked after the major issues: post-operative recovery, stitches and dressings, and preventing infection, but the business of physical appearance, mobility and emotional adjustment were left to the patient. So many new questions came up.

About this time a volunteer from the American Cancer Society's "Reach to Recovery" program showed up. Cheerful and healthy, the women who volunteer have to be at least one year post-mastectomy and have the recommendation of two doctors. They are living proof that one will eventually get out of bed and return to an active life. The volunteers are carefully trained to answer the "nuts and bolts" questions about mastectomy. They come armed with a kit courtesy of the American Cancer Society which contains a soft prosthesis and a loose-fitting bra so the patient can go home without the problem of clothes fitting strangely. Other items in the kit are a list of places locally where the patient can go to find a permanent prosthesis, booklets on care of the arm and hand, a rubber ball which one squeezes to help prevent

swelling in the affected arm, and a booklet of exercises on⟨
do to increase mobility of the shoulder joint and regain str⟨
in the arm. Most importantly the volunteer listens and
positive advice for coping with this new and confusing situa⟨

This service is invaluable to the post-op patient. It pro⟨
hope and the feeling that the patient has very specific thing⟨
can do to help herself recover. The information and su⟨
given by this program was a very important part o⟨
convalescence.

In the early days of cancer treatment I sometimes felt
alone and frightened. Having a friendly survivor to talk to ⟨
a big difference. I am so grateful to the American Cancer Sc⟨
for offering this worthwhile program.

PAT BRACK